AF691627

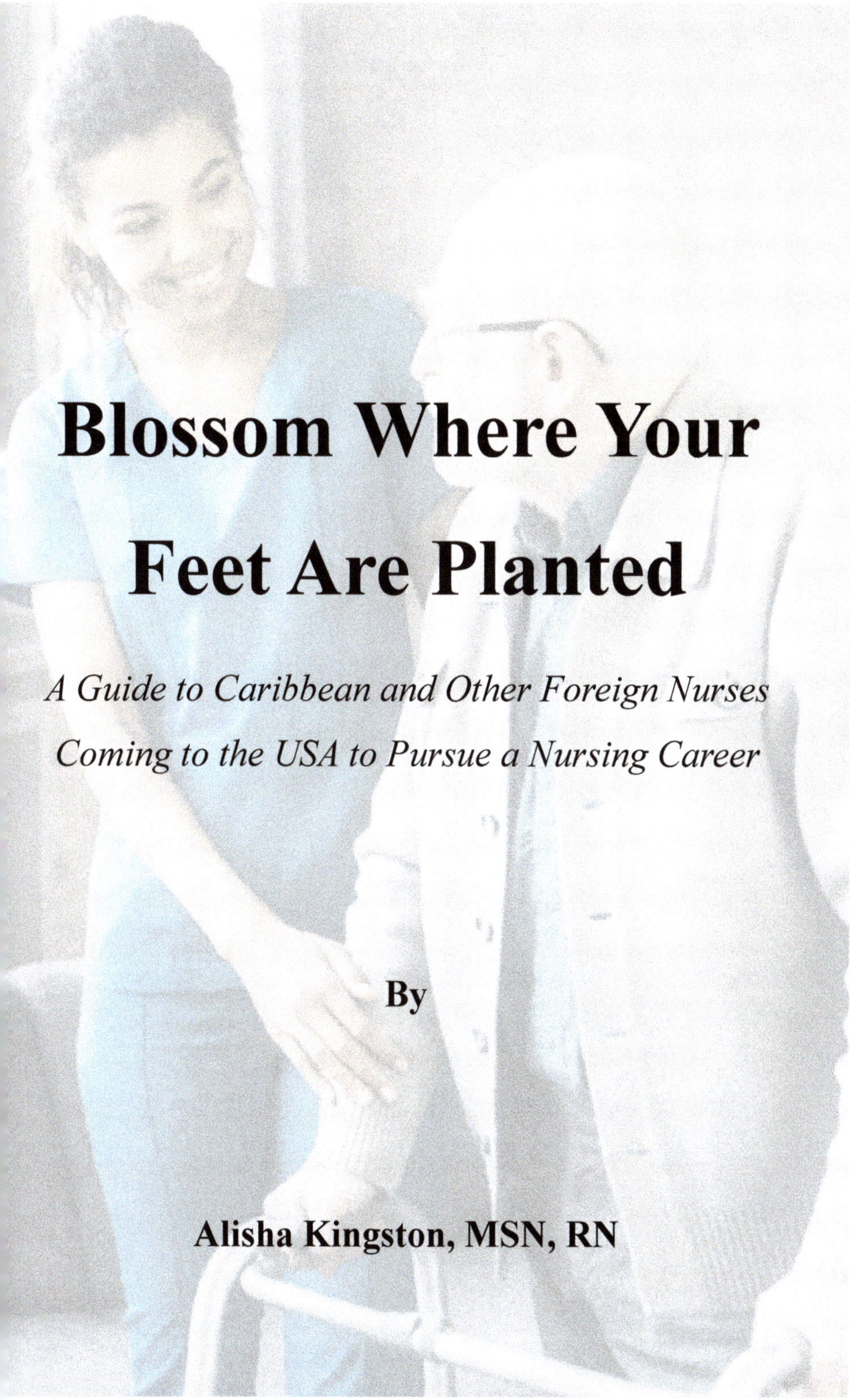

# Blossom Where Your Feet Are Planted

*A Guide to Caribbean and Other Foreign Nurses Coming to the USA to Pursue a Nursing Career*

**By**

**Alisha Kingston, MSN, RN**

Copyright © 2025 Alisha Kingston

All Rights Reserved.

No part of this work may be reproduced, distributed, or transmitted without prior written permission.

# Introduction

The composition of this book was driven by a deep desire to help other nurses who are new to the USA and in need of direction or guidance on how to restart their nursing careers. When I first arrived in the United States, I longed for someone who could guide me and show me the steps I needed to take. I reached out to others in the nursing field who had come before me, but unfortunately, I did not receive much help. With the support of my husband, I began researching the process myself and eventually learned how to resume my nursing career, specifically in North Carolina.

I decided that if I could help even a few nurses understand where to begin when they arrive, I would feel fulfilled. This book is my way of giving back, sharing my journey and the knowledge I gained in the hope that it makes someone else's path smoother. Whether you came to the USA through a nursing agency on a work visa or immigrated independently to take up permanent residence, having a healthy transition into the U.S. nursing profession is essential. It ensures not only a successful career but also the ability to contribute meaningfully to the American healthcare system.

# Acknowledgement

I would like to thank everyone who played a part in the development of my nursing career, those who guided my career choices and those who supported me emotionally, financially, and mentally. God is my guide, my strength, and my shield; all my success and happiness are because of Him.

Special thanks to my husband, Samuel Kingston, who has been and continues to be a source of unwavering support, a pillar of strength, and a true gift from God. Your encouragement, determination, support, and love are beyond words.

Our precious children, Olivia and Samuel, are a constant source of encouragement and motivation for us to keep moving forward. My parents, Anita and Basil Thomas, and my sisters, Vanessa Thomas-Bissoon and Nicola Thomas, supported me every step of the way with their hard work, encouragement, and love.

I am also grateful to my nursing tutors, lecturers, and counselors at Charles Rosa School of Nursing and Grand Canyon University. To my Seventh-day Adventist church families throughout the years, and to all other friends, colleagues, and relatives who have supported me, I thank you sincerely for all you have done.

This book is dedicated to all of you.

# Table of Contents

# Chapter 1: Background of My Profession Why I Chose It

Do not give up on your dreams, for dreams bring vision, vision brings hope and drive, and hope and drive can create your reality.

I grew up not knowing great earthly riches or wealth but came from a very humble beginning. With the encouragement of a close-knit family, supportive parents, an especially prayerful and strong mother, and of course, God, I always knew I had to do my best—to build myself, achieve my goals, and make them proud. I worked diligently from primary school through high school and nursing school. It was not always easy, especially financially, but sometimes all you need is perseverance, strength, hope, a persistent spirit, and a positive attitude. I found joy in reading, serving at church, and simply enjoying time with my family.

I always knew I wanted to be in the medical field, not only because I wanted to help those in need but also because of a very personal reason. I grew up watching my older sister suffer seizure after seizure. I saw my parents struggle to care for her and how challenging it was, especially for my mother. It deeply affected me because I often felt helpless, and I hated to see her suffer. I longed to know how I could help her better. By the time, I ventured into my medical career, she had stopped having seizures completely, but that did not stop my drive.

Initially, my dream was to become a medical doctor. While in high school, I applied for a Cuban scholarship to fulfill that goal. Although I was accepted in 2010, my parents preferred that I attend nursing school since it was closer to home. I chose to make them happy and enrolled in nursing instead. At first, I was not particularly fascinated, though I was not disappointed either—it was still in the medical field. My mind remained set on becoming a medical doctor someday. Nevertheless, I committed to the process of completing my nursing studies. I began in 2010, immediately after high school, and completed the program in 2014, earning a diploma in nursing. To my joy, I received the award for Best Graduating Clinical Registered Nurse. I was elated, and my professional journey officially began. I committed myself to offering the best nursing care I could.

After working for a year, in 2015 I pursued another opportunity to attend medical school and began studying at Georgetown American University on a partial scholarship. I was overwhelmed with joy, believing this must be what God intended for me since he opened another door. I performed well academically, but after a little over a year, life took an unexpected turn. At 23, I fell in love, married the most precious and caring man I know, and chose to move to the United States with him. It was one of the toughest decisions of my life, caught between a rock and a hard place, but it was also the best decision I ever made, and I have never looked back.

Coming to the USA brought new challenges, including obtaining my nursing license, having my education evaluated, preparing for the NCLEX, and deciding what direction my career should take. Part of me still debated whether to continue nursing or pursue medical school. However, once in the United States, I gained a new perspective. I realized the vast scope of nursing and saw my career in a different light. It solidified my decision to remain in nursing. I began to understand the truth in the statement: *nursing is the heart of healthcare.*

Before sitting for the NCLEX-RN, I also obtained a license as a registered pharmacy technician, which strengthened my pharmaceutical knowledge. I worked briefly as a home health aide, which gave me valuable insight into how nursing operates in the U.S. After obtaining my nursing license, I began working as a registered nurse—first in home health, then in infusion nursing. In less than a year, I secured my first hospital position. Realizing the importance of advancing my education to provide better care, I pursued my Bachelor of Science in Nursing at Grand Canyon University (GCU).

After completing my bachelor's degree, I recognized the value of lifelong learning and began my Master's in Nursing with an emphasis in Nursing Leadership in Healthcare Systems. This program helped me develop my leadership skills and broaden my vision for the future. During this time, I also began researching the terminal degrees in nursing—Doctor of Nursing Practice (DNP) and PhD—which opened a new world of possibilities for me. I set my sights on pursuing a DNP as a personal goal.

Looking back, I feel truly satisfied, overjoyed, and blessed by the steps I have taken to reach this point. It has been a privilege to touch the lives of others, whether directly or indirectly, through nursing. Nursing will forever hold a special place in my heart. I am currently working on completing my Family Nurse Practitioner program.

There is a quote from the legendary American basketball player Kobe Bryant that continues to inspire me: *"Those times when you stay up late and you work hard; those times when you don't feel like working, you're too tired, you don't feel like pushing yourself, but you do it anyway—that is actually the dream. It's not the destination. It's the journey."*

# Chapter 2: Coming to the USA

Coming to the USA presented me with several cultural shocks and professional readjustments. I faced my fair share of challenges along the way. This chapter will include the steps I took to obtain my U.S. nursing license:

- The transcript transfer process
- The CGFNS evaluation process
- The English proficiency exam
- Other agencies used by different states
- The nursing board process and involvement

What follows is a clear, structured guide with essential information for foreign-educated nurses coming to the USA, along with adjustment tips and insights on cultural shock awareness.

## 1. Professional & Licensing Requirements

- Credential Evaluation: Most states require verification of your nursing education (e.g., through CGFNS or ECE).
- English Proficiency: Unless you were educated in an English-speaking country, you will likely need to pass the TOEFL, IELTS, or PTE Academic.
- NCLEX-RN Exam: This mandatory national exam is required to obtain licensure. Prepare thoroughly, as the question style differs from other countries.

- State Variations: Each state board of nursing has its own rules regarding fees, forms, fingerprinting, and background checks. Research your chosen state early.
- Visa & Work Authorization: Common pathways include H-1B visas, EB-3 immigrant visas, or sponsorship through hospitals and recruiters.

## 2. Workplace Culture & Nursing Practice Differences

- Patient-Centered Care: Strong emphasis on patient autonomy and informed consent.
- Scope of Practice: Nurses often have broader responsibilities, including medication administration, care planning, and patient education.
- Technology Use: Expect to work with electronic health records (EHRs), medication scanning, and advanced monitoring systems.
- Team Dynamics: Collaboration with physicians, nurse practitioners, social workers, and therapists is routine.
- Documentation: Extremely detailed—if it's not documented, it didn't happen.

## 3. Adjustment & Cultural Shock

Moving to the USA can bring excitement but also emotional and cultural challenges.

**Common Cultural Shocks:**

- Communication Styles: Patients may be direct, ask many questions, or even challenge medical decisions.
- Diversity: You will care for patients from a wide range of cultural, religious, and ethnic backgrounds. Cultural competence is expected.
- Hierarchy Differences: Nurses are highly respected in the USA and are often more independent than in other countries.
- Lifestyle Adjustments: Food, climate, and daily routines may differ significantly from what you are used to at home.
- Workload & Pace: Nursing in the U.S. can be fast-paced, with high patient loads, especially in hospital settings.

**Coping Strategies:**

- Stay Open-Minded: Approach differences with curiosity rather than judgment.
- Build Support Networks: Join nursing associations (e.g., ANA, NCSBN, minority nurse groups) or local cultural communities.
- Ask Questions: It is normal to seek clarification on workplace policies and practices.
- Take Care of Your Mental Health: Culture shock often occurs in stages (honeymoon, frustration, adjustment, acceptance). Recognizing the cycle can help you manage it.

- Continue Learning: Participate in hospital orientations, professional development workshops, and cultural sensitivity training.

## 4. Daily Living in the USA

- Cost of Living: Varies widely between states and cities (e.g., New York vs. Texas). Research carefully before relocating.
- Banking & Finances: You will need a U.S. bank account, a credit history, and possibly an international money transfer setup.
- Healthcare System: Even as a nurse, you will need personal health insurance.
- Transportation: Public transit is limited in many cities, so having a driver's license and car may be essential.
- Community Integration: Volunteer, join professional groups, and participate in local events to feel more at home.

## 5. Success Tips for a Smooth Transition

- Be Patient with Yourself: Adjustment takes time.
- Celebrate Small Wins: Whether it's your first successful patient handoff or the first compliment from a patient, acknowledge your progress.
- Learn American Idioms and Slang: This will make communication smoother with both patients and coworkers.
- Maintain Ties with Family and Friends Back Home: Staying connected provides emotional support.

- Remember: Feeling “different” is normal; with time, you will gain confidence and adapt.

## Final Note

Coming to the USA as a nurse is both a professional achievement and a life-changing journey. The transition can feel overwhelming at times, but with preparation, support, and resilience, you can thrive both personally and professionally.

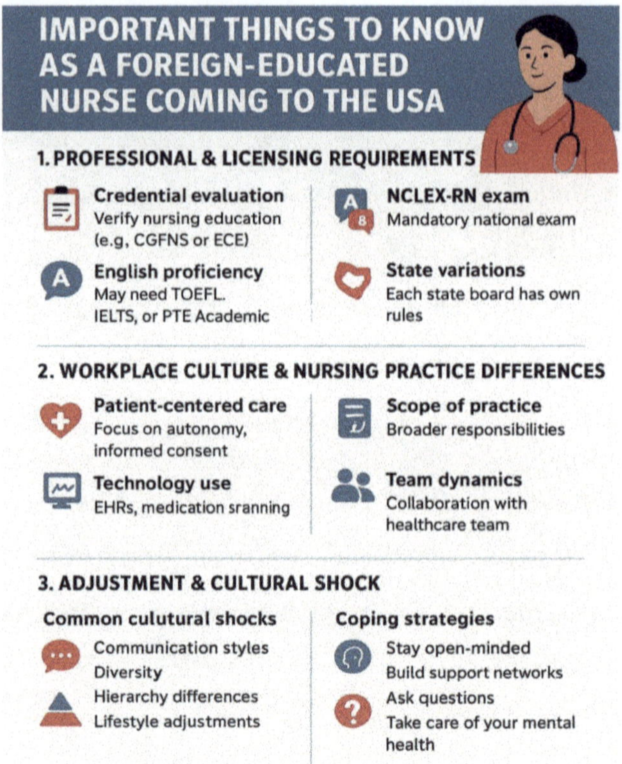

# Chapter 3: The NCLEX Experience

Quick Tip: I strongly advise starting your studies and making the necessary preparations as soon as you know you will be moving to the USA. Do not wait until after you arrive. This will help prevent delays between your arrival and the time you are ready to sit for the NCLEX-RN and obtain your license.

Preparing for the NCLEX-RN as a foreign-educated nurse can feel overwhelming, but with the right study resources, you will feel more confident and prepared. Here is a curated list of the most important and helpful study tools for you:

**Core NCLEX Prep Books**

**Saunders Comprehensive Review for the NCLEX-RN Examination (latest edition)**

- The gold standard review book, very detailed and covers all content areas.
- Includes practice questions and online resources.

**Kaplan NCLEX-RN Prep Plus**

- Excellent for strategies, test-taking skills, and critical thinking.
- Focuses on how to answer questions, not just on content.

**Lippincott Q&A Review for NCLEX-RN**

- Features more than 6,000 practice questions with detailed rationales.

**Mosby's Comprehensive Review of Nursing for the NCLEX-RN**

- Concise explanations and tons of practice questions.

**Online Question Banks (Qbanks)**

1. UWorld NCLEX-RN (Most recommended!)
   Realistic exam-style questions, detailed rationales, and performance tracking.
2. Kaplan Qbank
   Good for practicing test-taking strategies and prioritization.
3. Nurse Achieve
   AI-based adaptive testing (similar to the real NCLEX).
4. SimpleNursing.com
   Great for visual learners, short videos and mnemonics.

**Video & Visual Learning**

1. Simple Nursing (YouTube & website)
   Animated lessons, simplifies complex topics.
2. RegisteredNurseRN (YouTube)
   Free, clear explanations, practice quizzes, and tips.
3. Picmonic
   Uses cartoons and mnemonics to help memorize key facts.
4. Nursing.com (formerly NRSNG)
   Courses, videos, practice questions, and an NCLEX simulator.

**Mobile Apps for On-the-Go Review**

1. NCLEX RN Mastery (iOS/Android)

   Flashcards, practice questions, and daily reminders.

2. UWorld App

   Access to Qbank on your phone.

3. Picmonic App

   Quick visual mnemonics for memorization.

4. ATI RN Mentor

   Practice quizzes and rationales.

**Free Resources**

1. NCLEX Test Plan (from NCSBN) → Always review this!

   Outlines exactly what topics the exam covers.

   Link: ncsbn.org

2. NCSBN Learning Extension (NCSBN Review Course)

   Made by the creators of the NCLEX.

3. Quizlet Flashcards

   Thousands of user-made NCLEX decks.

**Special Tips for Foreign-Educated Nurses**

- Focus on U.S. Nursing Standards → Especially patient safety, prioritization, and legal/ethical guidelines, which may differ from your home country.
- Practice Select-All-That-Apply (SATA) → These are very common and tricky.

- Strengthen Medical English → Read U.S.-based nursing material to get used to terminology.
- Join Facebook/WhatsApp Study Groups → Many groups exist for international NCLEX test-takers. Many free resources are available in NCLEX Facebook groups (file/ folder section).

**Study Strategy Suggestion:**

*Start with Saunders (content review)*

- Review your school notes as needed, they are absolutely important and useful too.
- Practice daily with UWorld or any other question bank of your choice (questions + rationales).
- Use videos/mnemonics (SimpleNursing, Picmonic, RegisteredNurseRN) for reinforcement.
- Take 2–3 full-length practice exams under timed conditions.

Here's a structured 12-week (3-month) NCLEX study plan tailored for foreign-educated nurses, using the best mix of resources I listed earlier. It balances content review, practice questions, and test-taking strategies so you're ready and confident.

## 3-Month NCLEX Study Plan guide

### Month 1 – Build Your Foundation (Weeks 1–4)

Focus: Content Review + Building Confidence

***Daily Routine (4–6 hours):***

1. Content Review (Saunders / Nursing.com / SimpleNursing videos) → 2–3 hrs
2. UWorld Qbank Practice (40–50 questions/day) → 1.5–2 hrs

   Review all rationales (right & wrong answers).
3. Quick Mnemonics/Flashcards (Picmonic/Quizlet) → 30 mins

***Weekly Breakdown:***

Week 1–2: Fundamentals, Safety & Infection Control, Basic Care, Pharmacology basics

Week 3–4: Medical-Surgical (Cardiac, Respiratory, Neuro, Endocrine, GI, GU)

At the end of each week: Take a mini quiz (75–100 questions) to check progress.

**Month 2 – Practice & Application (Weeks 5–8)**

Focus: Applying knowledge + Prioritization/SATA practice

***Daily Routine (5–6 hours):***

1. Content Review (target weak areas) → 1–2 hrs
2. UWorld Qbank (60–75 questions/day) → 2–3 hrs

   Focus on SATA, delegation, prioritization, and infection control.
3. Test-taking Strategies (Kaplan book / RN Mastery app) → 30 mins
4. Mnemonics & Review (Picmonic/RegisteredNurseRN) → 30 mins

***Weekly Breakdown:***

Week 5–6: Maternal-Newborn Nursing & Pediatrics

Week 7–8: Psychiatric Nursing, Leadership/Management, Legal & Ethical

End of Week 6 & Week 8: Take a full-length 75–145 question simulated exam (UWorld or NurseAchieve).

**Month 3 – Mastery & Exam Readiness (Weeks 9–12)**

Focus: Exam Simulation & Weak Area Fixes

***Daily Routine (5–7 hours):***

1. Full-length Practice Exam (alternate days) → 75–145 questions Simulate real NCLEX conditions (quiet room, timed).
2. Detailed Review of Rationales → 2–3 hrs
3. Quick Content Refresh (Saunders summaries/flashcards) → 1 hr
4. Stress Management (short breaks, meditation, light exercise)

***Weekly Breakdown:***

Week 9–10: Rotate all subjects, focus on weaknesses shown in Qbank analytics.

Week 11: 2–3 full-length practice exams, review weak areas daily.

Week 12 (Final Week):

- 2 practice tests (early in week, not day before exam).
- Light review of high-yield topics:
- Pharmacology (must-know drugs, side effects, antidotes)

- Infection control (isolation precautions)
- Prioritization & delegation (who the nurse sees first, what task to delegate)
- Emergency/critical care (CPR, ABCs, safety first)

**Day Before Exam:**

- Rest, light review only.
- Avoid heavy studying.
- Sleep early.

**Additional Success Tips**

- Stick to U.S. guidelines (sometimes different from your home country).
- Practice SATA daily (they're ~30% of NCLEX).
- Read rationales carefully → Even when you get the answer right.
- Track progress → Use UWorld or Kaplan analytics to see weak areas.
- Simulate exam pressure → Take tests in one sitting, no distractions.

With this plan, you'll cover all NCLEX test plan areas, strengthen weak spots, and build exam stamina.

**Additional tips on how I studied:**

I selected a few good resources that work best for me and stick to those. Too many resources can be confusing to navigate through and can become overwhelming. I tried to keep it as simple as possible when studying. The resources I utilize include:

- RegisterednurseRN YouTube videos
- Mark Klimek audios (I listened to these on the Spotify app). These are so helpful during busy periods, for example, whilst you are cleaning or driving, you can still learn on the go by listening to these audios. He provides quality need to know nursing knowledge and NCLEX preparation tips in his audios.
- Facebook NCLEX pages resources in the file section are filled with an extensive amount of free NCLEX prep resources that can be accessed and used to improve the preparation experience. Many of those files can be accessed via the file section on those pages.
- Refresh my knowledge with my notebooks and textbooks, which I used in nursing school in Guyana. Don't turn your back on the information received during your nursing school journey; they are just as useful.

# Chapter 4: Let's Discuss Multistate License

Let's break this down step by step so you fully understand the Compact / Multistate Nursing License (NLC or eNLC) in the USA, how it works, the benefits, how to apply, and which states participate.

**What is a Compact or Multistate License?**

The Nurse Licensure Compact (NLC), also called the Enhanced Nurse Licensure Compact (eNLC), is an agreement between participating U.S. states that allows Registered Nurses (RNs) and Licensed Practical/Vocational Nurses (LPNs/LVNs) to have one license with the privilege to practice in multiple states.

Instead of applying for a new license every time you move or want to work in another participating state, you can practice freely across all compact states with just one multistate license.

**Important**

1. APRNs (Nurse Practitioners, CRNAs, CNMs, CNSs) are not included in the NLC. They must apply separately in each state.
2. Only nurses whose primary state of residence (PSOR) is a compact state can be issued a multistate license.

**Benefits of a Compact (Multistate) License**

1. **Work Across Multiple States**

Travel nurses, telehealth nurses, and nurses residing near state borders tend to benefit the most. Example: If you live in Texas, you can work in Florida, North Carolina, or any other compact state without needing to reapply.

2. **Faster Job Opportunities**

No waiting months for license endorsement. This is especially helpful for crisis response (e.g., pandemics, disasters).

3. **Cost-Effective**

Avoids multiple license application and renewal fees.

4. **Flexibility in Relocation**

If you move permanently to another compact state, you simply update your license to that new state.

5. **Telehealth Expansion**

You can provide telehealth nursing services across state lines without separate licenses.

**Current Compact States (as of August 2025)**

***Here's a list of states that participate in the eNLC:***

***Participating States (active):***

1. Alabama
2. Arizona

3. Arkansas
4. Colorado
5. Delaware
6. Florida
7. Georgia
8. Idaho
9. Indiana
10. Iowa
11. Kansas
12. Kentucky
13. Louisiana
14. Maine
15. Maryland
16. Mississippi
17. Missouri
18. Montana
19. Nebraska
20. New Hampshire
21. New Jersey (partial implementation, RNs/LPNs can apply for multistate privileges)
22. New Mexico
23. North Carolina
24. North Dakota
25. Ohio

26. Oklahoma
27. Pennsylvania (recently implemented)
28. South Carolina
29. South Dakota
30. Tennessee
31. Texas
32. Utah
33. Virginia
34. West Virginia
35. Wisconsin
36. Wyoming

***Not yet Compact States (require individual licensing):***

1. California
2. Connecticut
3. District of Columbia (DC)
4. Hawaii
5. Illinois
6. Massachusetts
7. Michigan
8. Minnesota
9. Nevada
10. New York
11. Oregon
12. Rhode Island

13. Washington
14. Vermont

Note: this list is subject to changes, so please research to see if there is a more updated list when you are about to start this process.

**Key Takeaways**

- The Compact License = one license, multiple states.
- Only available to RNs and LPNs/LVNs (not APRNs).
- You must live in a compact state to be eligible.
- Saves time, money, and effort, especially for travel nurses and telehealth.
- Over 40 states are now part of the compact, but large states like California and New York are still non-compact.

# Chapter 5: General Steps When Coming to Any State

Here's a detailed step-by-step outline of the general process a foreign-educated nurse (FEN) must follow to legally work as a registered nurse (RN) in the United States.

1. **Meet Basic Eligibility Requirements**

- Hold a nursing degree or diploma from an accredited nursing program outside the U.S.
- Be licensed as a nurse in your home country.
- Ensure your nursing education is comparable to U.S. standards (minimum of an associate degree in nursing, though most U.S. RNs hold a bachelor's degree).

2. **Credential Evaluation**

- Submit your nursing education and license for review through a recognized credentialing body, such as:
    - CGFNS International (Commission on Graduates of Foreign Nursing Schools)
    - Educational Records Evaluation Service (ERES) or other state-approved agencies

The evaluation verifies:

- Educational equivalency

- Nursing coursework and clinical hours
- Licensure authenticity

Some states require the **CGFNS Certification Program**, which includes:

- Credential verification
- Passing the CGFNS Qualifying Exam
- English proficiency testing (if applicable)

**3. English Language Proficiency (if applicable)**

If your nursing education was not in English, you must pass an English test such as:

- TOEFL (Test of English as a Foreign Language)
- IELTS (International English Language Testing System)
- TOEIC (Test of English for International Communication)

*Exemptions:* Nurses from English-speaking countries (e.g., UK, Canada, Australia) may be exempt, depending on the state.

**4. Apply for State Licensure**

Nursing is regulated at the state level, so you must apply to the Board of Nursing (BON) in the state where you plan to work.

The BON will review your:

- Credentials (CGFNS or equivalent)
- English proficiency results
- Background check/fingerprints

5. **Register for the NCLEX-RN Exam**

Once approved by the state BON, you will be eligible to take the NCLEX-RN (National Council Licensure Examination for Registered Nurses).

***Steps:***

1. Apply through Pearson VUE (the testing company).
2. Receive your Authorization to Test (ATT).
3. Schedule and take the exam.

Passing the NCLEX is mandatory to become a licensed RN in the U.S.

6. **Obtain Visa and Immigration Clearance**

To work as a nurse in the U.S., you must have a legal work visa.

**Common options:**

- **EB-3 Visa (Employment-Based Green Card for Skilled Workers)**
    - Most popular for foreign nurses
    - Requires employer sponsorship
- **H-1B Visa (Specialty Occupations)** – less common for nurses but possible in advanced roles (e.g., nurse practitioners)

CGFNS issues the **VisaScreen Certificate**, which U.S. immigration requires to verify:

- Credentials

- English proficiency
- NCLEX (or equivalent exam) passage

7. **Secure Employment**

- Apply for RN positions with hospitals, clinics, or healthcare facilities.
- Many U.S. hospitals and staffing agencies actively recruit foreign nurses.
- Your employer may sponsor your visa/green card process.

8. **Relocate and Begin Practice**

Upon arrival in the U.S., complete:

- State-specific licensing requirements (some states require additional orientation or training)
- Employment onboarding at your healthcare facility

9. **Maintain and Renew Your License**

- Nurses must renew their licenses periodically (every 2–3 years, depending on the state).
- Renewal typically requires continuing education (CEU) credits.

**Quick Summary Checklist**

- Nursing degree + license in home country (remember all transcripts sent to CGFNS need to be directly from your nursing school, not from you. CGFNS only accepts sealed transcripts and other documents from the specific agency it was prepared by.

- Credential evaluation (CGFNS or state-approved)
- English proficiency test (if required)
- Apply for state BON licensure
- Pass NCLEX-RN
- Obtain VisaScreen certificate
- Secure U.S. employer & visa sponsorship
- Relocate and begin working
- Maintain license

1. A general roadmap with estimated timelines (so you can see how long each step usually takes).
2. A state-by-state comparison chart (focusing on major states where foreign nurses often apply).

**General Roadmap for Foreign Nurses Coming to the U.S.**

| Step | What You Do | Estimated Time |
|---|---|---|
| Credential Evaluation (CGFNS or equivalent) | Submit transcripts, license verification, and education records. | 3–6 months |
| English Proficiency Exam (if required) | Take TOEFL/IELTS/TOEIC. | 1–2 months (prep + results) |
| Apply to State Board of Nursing (BON) | Choose the state where you want to work and submit your application. | 2–4 months (varies by state) |
| Register for NCLEX-RN | Apply through Pearson VUE and get Authorization to Test (ATT). | 1–2 months |
| Take and Pass NCLEX-RN | Required for licensure. | 1–2 months (depends on exam scheduling) |

| | | |
|---|---|---|
| Obtain VisaScreen | Certificate CGFNS verifies credentials, English, and NCLEX results. | 3–4 months |
| Secure Employer | Sponsorship Hospital/agency files petition for EB-3 or other visa. | 6–12 months (green card process may take longer depending on the country) |
| Relocate to the U.S. | Enter the U.S. and begin employment. | After visa approval |
| License Renewal & Continuing Education | Renew license every 2–3 years (varies by state). | Ongoing |

Average total time: 1.5–3 years (faster if paperwork is prepared early and employer sponsorship is quick).

**State-by-State Comparison (Foreign Nurse Licensure)**

Here's a simplified list for popular states where many international nurses apply:

Order for description: State, Credential Evaluation Required, CGFNS Exam Required? English Test Required? Additional Notes

**New York (NY)**

- **Credential Evaluation:** Yes (CGFNS/NYSED-approved agency)
- **CGFNS Exam Required:** No (only evaluation)
- **English Proficiency:** Yes (if non-English program)
- **Notes:** One of the most foreign-nurse-friendly states; no CGFNS exam required.

**California (CA)**

- **Credential Evaluation:** Yes (Board-approved evaluation)

- **CGFNS Exam Required:** No
- **English Proficiency:** Yes (unless English program)
- **Notes:** California has strict rules about clinical hours, which must match U.S. standards.

**Texas (TX)**

- **Credential Evaluation:** Yes (via CGFNS CES Report)
- **CGFNS Exam Required:** No
- **English Proficiency:** Yes
- **Notes:** The BON is usually fast but requires fingerprints and a background check.

**Florida (FL)**

- **Credential Evaluation:** Yes (via CGFNS CES Report)
- **CGFNS Exam Required:** No
- **English Proficiency:** Yes
- **Notes:** Accepts CES plus NCLEX; popular choice for international nurses.

**Illinois (IL)**

- **Credential Evaluation:** Yes (CGFNS or equivalent)
- **CGFNS Exam Required:** Yes (CGFNS exam required)
- **English Proficiency:** Yes
- **Notes:** One of the few states that still requires the CGFNS qualifying exam.

**New Jersey (NJ)**

- **Credential Evaluation:** Yes (CES Report)
- **CGFNS Exam Required:** No
- **English Proficiency:** Yes
- **Notes:** Straightforward process; VisaScreen still needed for immigration.

**Michigan (MI)**

- **Credential Evaluation:** Yes (CES Report)
- **CGFNS Exam Required:** No
- **English Proficiency:** Yes
- **Notes:** Requires a Social Security Number for final license issuance.

**Texas, Florida, and New York**

- **Status:** Known as international nurse hubs
- **CGFNS Exam Required:** No
- **Notes:** Often preferred due to faster BON processing.

Tip: If you want the fastest path, states like New York, Texas, and Florida are usually more friendly for foreign nurses (no CGFNS exam required, just NCLEX + credential eval).

Caution: States like Illinois or Vermont may slow the process due to requiring the CGFNS Qualifying Exam.

## STEPS CGFNS TAKES TO TRANSCRIBE/ VERIFY A FOREIGN-EDUCATED NURSE'S CREDENTIALS

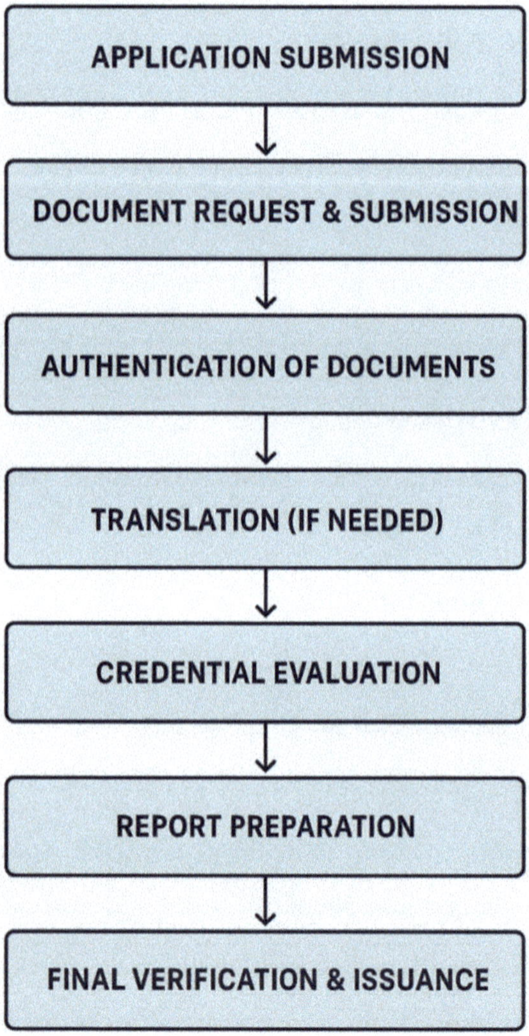

# Chapter 6: Credentialing Bodies in the USA for Verification of Foreign-Educated Nurses Certification

In the U.S., several credentialing bodies are authorized to evaluate and verify foreign-educated nurses' credentials for state boards of nursing and sometimes for immigration. Each state board decides which agency it accepts. Here's a breakdown:

1. **CGFNS International (Commission on Graduates of Foreign Nursing Schools)**

Most widely recognized and accepted by the majority of U.S. states.

*Services:*

- CES (Credentials Evaluation Service)
- CVS for New York State (required only by NY)
- Certification Program
- VisaScreen (for immigration)

*States that specifically mandate CGFNS:*

- New York → requires CVS (CGFNS is the only provider accepted).
- Michigan, New Jersey, Pennsylvania, and others often specify CGFNS for CES or Certification.

- Widely accepted nationwide by boards of nursing, employers, and USCIS.

2. **Josef Silny & Associates, Inc. (JS&A)**

- An independent credential evaluation service.
- Accepted by some state boards of nursing.

*States that accept JS&A:*

- Florida BON (lists JS&A as an approved credentialing agency).
- May also be accepted in certain other states that allow multiple evaluation agencies.

3. **Educational Records Evaluation Service (ERES)**

- Based in Sacramento, California.
- Performs nursing credential evaluations for U.S. boards.

*States that accept ERES:*

- California Board of Registered Nursing (BRN) accepts ERES for transcript evaluation.
- Sometimes accepted in Oregon and other western states.

4. **International Education Research Foundation (IERF)**

- One of the oldest evaluation agencies in the U.S.
- Provides course-by-course evaluations for nurses.

*States that accept IERF:*

- California Board of Registered Nursing (BRN) accepts IERF for foreign nursing credentials.
- Accepted in Texas for certain categories of nursing applicants.

5. **Educational Credential Evaluators (ECE)**

- Provides course-by-course and document-by-document evaluations.
- Not as nursing-specific as CGFNS but accepted by some boards.

*States that accept ECE:*

- The Texas BON accepts ECE for foreign-educated nurses.
- Other states may allow ECE if they accept multiple credential evaluators.

**Summary by State Requirements**

- Exclusive CGFNS requirement: New York (CVS program), many Northeastern states.
- California: Accepts ERES or IERF (not CGFNS for initial RN licensing, except for VisaScreen immigration purposes).
- Florida: Accepts JS&A as well as CGFNS.
- Texas: Accepts ECE, IERF, and CGFNS.
- Other states: Vary — some only list CGFNS, others allow multiple approved evaluators.

**Key takeaway:**

- CGFNS is the most widely accepted and sometimes the only option.
- California, Texas, and Florida stand out for recognizing other evaluators (IERF, ERES, JS&A, ECE).

- Nurses must always check their state board of nursing's website for the approved list of credentialing agencies, since requirements differ significantly.

# Chapter 7: Job Seeking and Working

As a New USA Nurse: Surviving Your First Shift and Adapting in Your New Job

- **Get the most out of your mentor.** During orientation phase, your mentor or preceptor will be the most important person to you. Also, become familiar with other members of your team. You can learn so much more by networking with members of your unit team.
- **Stop complaining and remain calm.**
- **Observe the experts.**
- **Expect the worst but hold integrity.**

This is a huge step, and the U.S. healthcare system can feel overwhelming at first for foreign-educated registered nurses (RNs). Here's some practical, real-world advice to help you succeed:

1. **Be Strategic About Where You Apply**

- Target states friendly to foreign nurses: e.g., New York, Texas, Florida, New Jersey, which don't require the CGFNS Qualifying Exam and have high demand.
- Consider Nurse Licensure Compact (NLC) states — if you get licensed in one, you may work across multiple states without relicensing.

- Research hospitals and staffing agencies that are known to sponsor visas (EB-3 is the most common for nurses).

**2. Choose the Right Employer**

- Large hospital systems often have structured programs for international nurses (orientation, visa sponsorship, NCLEX support).
- Rural hospitals & long-term care facilities are more likely to sponsor visas quickly due to nursing shortages.
- Avoid employers/third-party recruiters that charge high fees or lock you into unfair contracts (some agencies bind nurses to 3–5 years with penalties for leaving early). Always read contracts carefully.

**Note:** In some states it is a bit more difficult to land a hospital job as a new USA RN with only foreign nursing experience. If this is the case for you, here are a few things you can do:

- Choose to volunteer in the hospital of your choice, if volunteer opportunities are available. Then seek to transfer into a full-time paid position.
- Check out travel nursing jobs in your local state or surrounding states, these usually have high demand for nurses giving you a better chance of getting hired in a hospital to gain experience to add to your resume. The biggest pro is that travel jobs pay well above the normal staff nurse receive. Additionally, you will be

able to enjoy travel experience. Many agencies will reimburse travel, provide meal allowances and other benefits.

- Try the old fashion method of actually going in to meet the nurse manager once you submit your application. This shows intent, giving you a better chance of getting hired.
- Keep applying, don't give up.
- Ensure you update your resume well and detailed and that it accurately reflects all your experiences. Include any volunteer work you have done that may be deemed necessary on your resume.

**3. Strengthen Your Resume & Application**

- Highlight international nursing experience — clinical specialties (ICU, ER, Med-Surg, Pediatrics, etc.).
- Translate nursing terminology into U.S. standards (e.g., say "Med-Surg" instead of "General Ward").
- Emphasize language proficiency and any U.S. certifications you've already earned (BLS, ACLS, PALS).

**4. Prepare for Interviews & Cultural Fit**

- U.S. hospitals value teamwork, communication, and adaptability as much as technical skill.
- Be ready to answer scenario-based questions (e.g., handling a difficult patient, prioritizing care for multiple patients).

- Learn about patient rights, HIPAA (privacy law), and documentation standards in the U.S.—interviewers often check for awareness of these.

5. **Understand Pay, Benefits & Cost of Living**

- RN salaries vary widely: $30–$60/hour depending on state and setting. Urban hospitals often pay more but have higher living costs.
- Check if the employer offers housing support, relocation assistance, or sign-on bonuses (common in shortage areas).
- Always confirm overtime policies and shift differentials (extra pay for nights/weekends).

6. **Secure the Right Visa & Legal Status**

- Most foreign nurses come under the EB-3 Green Card (Skilled Worker) visa, sponsored by an employer.
- While waiting, some work under temporary visas (rare and limited to advanced roles).
- You'll need a VisaScreen Certificate from CGFNS before your visa can be approved.

7. **Adapt to U.S. Workplace Culture**

- U.S. nursing practice is often more independent than in some countries—RNs make critical decisions and delegate tasks to CNAs or LPNs.

- Patient expectations: Americans often expect clear explanations of care and may challenge or question providers.
- Be proactive about continuing education (CEUs) to keep your license active.

**8. Build a Support Network**

- Join professional associations like the American Nurses Association (ANA) or state nursing associations.
- Connect with other foreign nurses through Facebook groups, LinkedIn, or local community organizations.
- Having a community helps with both career growth and personal adjustment.

**9. Think Long-Term**

- Once settled, you can pursue advanced nursing roles (e.g., Nurse Practitioner, Clinical Nurse Specialist) by furthering your education in the U.S.
- These roles often come with higher pay and greater autonomy, and some employers may help fund your education.
- Consider starting in shortage specialties (ICU, ER, geriatrics)—these areas have the highest demand and best job security.

**Key Takeaway**

Be selective with your employer, protect yourself from exploitative contracts, and aim for states/hospitals that support foreign nurses with mentorship and sponsorship. The U.S. system values not just your skills, but also communication, teamwork, and cultural adaptability.

- Ask questions and ask for help. It's totally fine not to know everything; in fact, even as a seasoned RN, you will never know everything.
- Bond with your new team.
- Understand when you need to recharge.
- Prioritize and time management.
- Invest time in continuing education.
- Self-care (Mental, emotional, spiritual and physical).
- Take advantage of professional organizations.
- Reassess yourself daily after your shift to understand what are your strengths and weaknesses.
- Don't be afraid to admit your mistakes. This is an important step to growing.
- Be open to new opportunities to make you grow; such as new assignments, new procedures, floating to another unit, volunteering.
- ***Ask pertinent questions when meeting with human resource and your manager: insurance coverage, nurse patient ratio, paid leave accrual, job description (ensure you familiarize yourself with this and always ensure you have access to a copy so you know your limitations and scope regarding your practice) sick leave policies, time off, read policies and***

***procedures guiding practice well, academic support, growth opportunities.***

Here's a solid list of trusted websites and platforms where foreign-educated nurses (and nurses in general) can utilize to apply for nursing jobs in the USA:

**General Job Boards (Healthcare-Focused and General)**

1. **Indeed** – indeed.com

   One of the largest job boards in the US. Thousands of nursing postings daily. Allows filtering by visa sponsorship or *"international nurses."*

2. **Glassdoor** – glassdoor.com

   Job listings + company reviews to help you evaluate employers. Great for checking salary expectations and work environment.

3. **ZipRecruiter** – ziprecruiter.com

   Widely used job portal with healthcare-specific postings.

4. **LinkedIn Jobs** – linkedin.com/jobs

   Excellent for networking with recruiters. Many hospitals and agencies hire directly via LinkedIn.

**Healthcare & Nursing-Specific Job Boards**

5. **Nurse.com** – nurse.com/jobs

   Nursing-specific jobs across the USA.

6. **NursingJobs.com** – nursingjobs.com

   Focused on RN, BSN, MSN, and specialty nursing roles.

7. **RN Network** – rnnetwork.com

   Travel nursing and permanent positions.

8. **TravelNurseSource** – travelnursesource.com

   Specializes in travel nurse positions, some offer sponsorship.

9. **American Nurses Association (ANA) Career Center** – nursingworld.org/jobs

   Listings from reputable healthcare systems nationwide.

**For Foreign-Educated / International Nurses**

10. **O'Grady Peyton International** – ogradypeyton.com

    A major agency helping international nurses migrate and work in the USA.

11. **Avant Healthcare Professionals** – avanthealthcare.com

    Specializes in recruiting international nurses, supports with NCLEX, visa, and relocation.

12. **Worldwide HealthStaff Solutions** – healthstaff.org

    Focuses on placing international nurses in permanent U.S. jobs.

13. **Conexus MedStaff** – conexusmedstaff.com

    Hires foreign nurses and helps with immigration & NCLEX preparation.

14. **ADEX Medical Staffing** – adexmedicalstaffing.com

    Works with international RNs and offers green card sponsorship.

**Government & Hospital Systems**

15. **USAJobs.gov** – usajobs.gov

    Official site for federal nursing jobs (Veterans Affairs, Department of Defense, Indian Health Service, etc.). Many federal hospitals hire international nurses with sponsorship.

16. **Major Health Systems' Career Pages** (apply directly for better chances):

    - **Mayo Clinic** – jobs.mayoclinic.org
    - **Cleveland Clinic** – jobs.clevelandclinic.org
    - **Johns Hopkins** – jobs.hopkinsmedicine.org
    - **HCA Healthcare** – careers.hcahealthcare.com

**Tips for International Nurses Applying Online**

- Use keywords like **"visa sponsorship," "international RN," or "foreign-educated nurse."**
- Tailor your resume to U.S. standards (clear formatting, NCLEX/English test status, credentials).
- Consider applying through staffing agencies that specialize in international nurses for higher success rates.

# Chapter 8: Understanding Nurse-to-Patient Ratio in the USA

The nurse-to-patient ratio is one of the biggest adjustments foreign-educated nurses notice when they begin practicing in the USA. Here's a breakdown of what to expect:

**1. No Federal Standard**

- The U.S. does not have a nationwide law for nurse-to-patient ratios.
- Ratios vary by state, hospital policy, unit type, and staffing availability.

**2. California: The Only State with Mandated Ratios**
California is the only state with legally mandated minimum staffing ratios:

- ICU: 1 nurse to 2 patients
- Emergency Room: 1 to 4
- Medical-Surgical Unit: 1 to 5
- Labor & Delivery: 1 to 2 for active labor

Other states may have staffing guidelines but no enforceable laws.

**3. Typical Ratios You May Encounter**

- ICU (Critical Care) → 1:1 or 1:2
- Step-Down / Progressive Care → 1:3–4

- Med-Surg (Medical-Surgical) → 1:5–7 (varies widely; in some places, it may stretch to 1:8)
- Emergency Department → 1:3–4, but can fluctuate during crises
- Labor & Delivery → 1:1 in active labor, 1:2 in postpartum
- Long-Term Care / Nursing Homes → Often higher ratios, e.g., 1 RN to 20+ residents, with LPNs and CNAs assisting

**4. What This Means for Foreign-Educated Nurses**

- Workload may feel heavier compared to some countries where staffing is stricter.
- Nurses are expected to manage time efficiently, use support staff (CNAs, techs, LPNs), and prioritize care.
- Documentation (charting) takes significant time — U.S. nurses spend 25–35% of their shifts on electronic health records.
- Safe practice and advocacy: If you feel unsafe with your assignment, you can escalate concerns to your charge nurse or nurse manager.

**5. What to Expect and How to Adapt**

- Be prepared for 12-hour shifts with multiple patients.
- Learn to delegate tasks (CNAs can help with vitals, hygiene, and feeding).
- Develop strong organizational and communication skills.

- Join professional associations (such as ANA or state nursing associations), many of which advocate for better ratios.

**Bottom Line**

A nurse coming to the USA should expect ratios that vary by unit and state, often heavier than in some countries. Strong teamwork, efficient charting, and self-advocacy are key to managing safely and effectively.

# Chapter 9: The Importance of a Good, Well-Structured & Up-to-Date Resume

A resume is more than just a list of qualifications; it is your professional first impression to potential employers. For foreign-educated nurses entering the U.S. healthcare system, the resume plays an even greater role in bridging cultural, educational, and professional differences.

**1. Showcases Transferable Skills and Global Experience**

- Many U.S. employers may not recognize nursing schools, hospitals, or health systems from abroad.
- A clear, structured resume highlights clinical expertise, certifications, and patient care experience in a way that translates to U.S. standards.
- Demonstrates how your international background adds diversity and adaptability to the healthcare team.

**2. Demonstrates Professionalism**

- Following U.S. formatting standards (chronological or hybrid, concise, achievement-focused) reassures employers that you are prepared for the American job market.
- Shows that you value organization, attention to detail, and presentation, qualities highly valued in nursing.

**3. Keeps You Competitive in a Highly Demanding Job Market**

- U.S. hospitals often receive hundreds of applications for a single nursing position.
- A strong resume immediately highlights:
  - Nursing license (RN/NCLEX)
  - Specialized skills
  - U.S. healthcare experience (if any)
- Outdated or poorly formatted resumes are often overlooked, even if the candidate is qualified.

**4. Reflects Career Growth and Continuing Education**

- U.S. nursing values lifelong learning (certifications, advanced practice, CEUs).
- Regularly updating your resume ensures new skills, workshops, and clinical rotations are recorded.
- Demonstrates professional growth and commitment to staying current.

**5. Supports Visa Sponsorship or Employer Requirements**

- Employers sponsoring foreign nurses often need to verify credentials quickly.
- A complete, updated resume speeds up HR processing for immigration and licensing compliance.

**6. Opens Doors to Specialization**

- If you're targeting a specialty (ICU, pediatrics, oncology, OR, etc.), your resume highlights relevant experience and certifications.
- U.S. nurses often pursue specialty certifications listing these shows initiative and ambition.

**7. Builds Confidence in Interviews**

- A polished resume not only impresses employers but also acts as a roadmap during interviews.
- Helps you recall accomplishments, clinical cases, and leadership experiences with ease.

**Quick Tips for Foreign-Educated Nurses**

- Keep your resume 1–2 pages.
- Clearly state your U.S. nursing license status (NCLEX passed, CGFNS certified, or in process).
- Highlight clinical skills, language abilities, and adapt your experience to U.S. healthcare terminology.

**Sample Resume Template – Foreign-Educated Nurse in the USA**

Full Name, RN, MSN (if applicable)

City, State | Phone Number | Email | LinkedIn (optional)

## Professional Summary

Compassionate and detail-oriented foreign-educated Registered Nurse with over 5 years of clinical experience in medical-surgical and critical care units. Recently licensed as a Registered Nurse in the United States after passing the NCLEX-RN. Skilled in patient-centered care, medication administration, and interdisciplinary collaboration. Bilingual in English and [your language], bringing cultural competence and adaptability to diverse patient populations.

## Licensure & Certifications

Registered Nurse (RN), [State], License #XXXXXX – Active, Expires [MM/YYYY]

NCLEX-RN – Passed [Year]

Basic Life Support (BLS), American Heart Association – Valid until [MM/YYYY]

Advanced Cardiovascular Life Support (ACLS) – Valid until [MM/YYYY]

[Any specialty certifications: e.g., Pediatric Advanced Life Support (PALS), CCRN, etc.]

## Education

Bachelor of Science in Nursing (BSN) – [School, Country], [Year]

Credential evaluated by CGFNS/approved educational evaluation agency – equivalent to U.S. BSN

[If applicable: MSN, ADN, Diploma Nursing, or current U.S. nursing program enrollment]

## Professional Experience

**Staff Nurse – Medical-Surgical Unit**

[Hospital Name, City, Country] | [MM/YYYY] – [MM/YYYY]

- Delivered patient care in a 20-bed medical-surgical unit with diverse patient populations.
- Monitored vital signs, administered medications, and assisted in diagnostic procedures.
- Educated patients and families on post-discharge care and chronic disease management.
- Collaborated with a multidisciplinary team to improve patient outcomes.

**Staff Nurse – Intensive Care Unit (ICU)**

[Hospital Name, City, Country] | [MM/YYYY] – [MM/YYYY]

- Provided critical care to patients requiring ventilator management, IV drips, and advanced monitoring.

- Assisted in emergency interventions such as Code Blue, rapid response, and intubations.
- Ensured compliance with infection control protocols and patient safety standards.

(Add additional roles if applicable; keep descriptions achievement-focused and concise.)

## Clinical Experience in the U.S. (if applicable)

### Observership / Preceptorship / Volunteer Nurse

[Hospital/Clinic Name, City, State] | [MM/YYYY] – [MM/YYYY]

- Shadowed registered nurses in [department/unit], gaining exposure to U.S. healthcare practices.
- Assisted with patient education and documentation under supervision.

## Skills

- Patient Assessment & Documentation
- Medication Administration (IV, IM, Oral)
- Electronic Health Records (Epic, Cerner – list if experienced)
- Infection Control & Patient Safety
- Interdisciplinary Teamwork
- Bilingual: English & [Language]

## Professional Affiliations (optional)

1. Member, American Nurses Association (ANA)
2. Member, [State] Nurses Association
3. Member, [Specialty Organization, e.g., AACN for Critical Care Nurses]

## Tips for Use

- Keep your resume 1–2 pages maximum.
- Use U.S. job titles (e.g., “Registered Nurse” instead of “Staff Nurse” if equivalent).
- Emphasize U.S. readiness: NCLEX, CGFNS, and state licensure.
- Tailor your summary and skills to match the job description.

# Chapter 10: Importance of Maintaining Certifications such as BLS, ACLS

Maintaining certifications such as Basic Life Support (BLS) and Advanced Cardiovascular Life Support (ACLS) is essential for nurses, as they demonstrate ongoing competence in critical, lifesaving skills. These certifications ensure that nurses are prepared to respond quickly and effectively in emergencies such as cardiac arrest, respiratory failure, or other life-threatening events. They also reflect professional accountability, since many employers and regulatory bodies require them for practice in acute care and specialty settings. Keeping certifications current enhances patient safety, boosts a nurse's confidence in high-stress situations, and strengthens career opportunities by meeting the standards of modern healthcare practice.

# IMPORTANCE OF MAINTAINING CERTIFICATIONS

**BLS**
BASIC LIFE SUPPORT

**ACLS**
ADVANCED CARDIOVASCULAR LIFE SUPPORT

## DEMONSTRATES ONGOING COMPETENCE

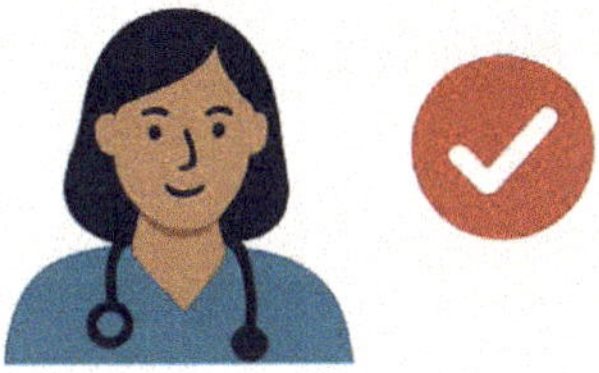

Ensures nurses ar prepred to respond quickly and effectively in emergencies

## REFLECTS PROFESSIONAL ACCOUNTABILITY

Many employers and regulatory bodies require them for practice

## ENHANCES PATIENT SAFETY

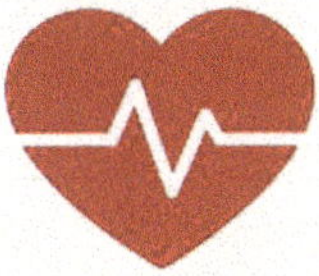

Boosts a nurse's confidence and ability to deliver life-saving interventions

## STRENGTHENS CAREER OPPORTUNITIES

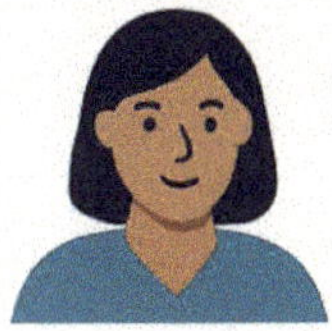

Meets the stantards of healthcare organizations and opens advancement opt-

Beyond Basic Life Support (BLS) and Advanced Cardiovascular Life Support (ACLS), different hospital departments and specialties often require or strongly recommend additional certifications. Here's a breakdown by department:

**Emergency Department (ED/ER)**

- **PALS (Pediatric Advanced Life Support):** Caring for critically ill or injured children
- **TNCC (Trauma Nursing Core Course):** Trauma patient assessment and interventions
- **ENPC (Emergency Nursing Pediatric Course):** Pediatric emergency care
- **CEN (Certified Emergency Nurse):** Advanced credential for ED nurses

**Pediatrics / NICU / PICU**

- **PALS (Pediatric Advanced Life Support):** Pediatric resuscitation
- **NRP (Neonatal Resuscitation Program):** Newborn stabilization
- **CPN (Certified Pediatric Nurse):** Pediatric nursing certification
- **RNC-NIC (Neonatal Intensive Care Nursing Certification):** NICU specialty

**Critical Care / ICU / CCU**

- **PCCN (Progressive Care Certified Nurse):** Step-down/progressive care patients
- **CCRN (Critical Care Registered Nurse):** Adult, pediatric, or neonatal ICU specialty
- **CSC (Cardiac Surgery Certification):** Open-heart surgery recovery units
- **CFRN (Certified Flight Registered Nurse):** For critical transport nursing

**Cardiac / Cath Lab / Telemetry**

- **ACLS:** Already required
- **CFRN or CTRN (Transport Nursing):** For cardiac transport
- **RCIS (Registered Cardiovascular Invasive Specialist):** Optional for RNs in the cath lab
- **PCCN or CCRN:** If working in step-down or ICU-level cardiac care

**Medical-Surgical / General Nursing**

- **CMSRN (Certified Medical-Surgical Registered Nurse):** Med-surg specialty
- **ONS/ONCC (Oncology Nursing Certification):** For caring for cancer patients
- **IV Therapy Certification:** State-dependent requirement

**Labor & Delivery / OB-GYN**

- **NRP (Neonatal Resuscitation Program):** Required in L&D and postpartum
- **AWHONN Fetal Monitoring:** Interpreting fetal heart monitoring
- **RNC-OB (Inpatient Obstetric Nursing Certification):** OB specialty
- **C-EFM (Electronic Fetal Monitoring Certification):** Fetal monitoring credential

**Psychiatric / Behavioral Health**

- **PMH-BC (Psychiatric-Mental Health Nursing Certification):** Psychiatric specialty
- **CPI (Crisis Prevention Intervention):** De-escalation and safety training

**Other Specialized Areas**

- **Burn Nursing:** ABLS (Advanced Burn Life Support)
- **Dialysis/Nephrology:** CDN (Certified Dialysis Nurse) or CNN (Certified Nephrology Nurse)
- **Oncology:** OCN (Oncology Certified Nurse)
- **Infection Control:** CIC (Certification in Infection Control)
- **OR/Perioperative:** CNOR (Certified Perioperative Nurse)

**Quick Tip for Foreign-Educated Nurses Transitioning to the USA**

Many hospitals sponsor training for required certifications once you're hired (especially PALS, NRP, and ACLS renewals). Specialty certifications like CCRN, CEN, or CMSRN usually require a certain number of practice hours before you are eligible.

# Chapter 11: Differences That Foreign Educated Nurses May Notice During Their Transition

Foreign-educated nurses often notice several key differences when they begin working in the USA. Some of the most common include:

1. **Automated and Electronic Systems**

   U.S. hospitals rely heavily on electronic health records (EHRs), barcoding systems, and automated medication-dispensing machines. Nurses may need to quickly adapt to the extensive use of technology for charting, order entry, and communication.

2. **Continuing Education (CEU) Requirements**

   In the U.S., nurses are required to complete Continuing Education Units (CEUs) for license renewal. CEU requirements vary by state, and courses can be taken online or in person to maintain competency and stay current with best practices.

3. **Scope of Practice Differences**

   The nursing scope of practice is regulated at the state level, meaning what nurses are allowed to do in one state may differ in another. For example, some states grant more autonomy to advanced practice nurses (like Nurse Practitioners), while others enforce stricter physician oversight requirements.

4. **Patient-Centered Care and Autonomy**

   Nurses in the U.S. often have greater autonomy in clinical decision-making compared to some countries. They actively participate in interdisciplinary teams and play a significant role in patient education.

5. **Legal and Documentation Standards**

   U.S. nursing practice places a strong emphasis on legal accountability and thorough documentation, as nursing notes are often used in audits, insurance claims, and even legal proceedings.

6. **Work Culture and Interdisciplinary Collaboration**

   Many U.S. healthcare facilities emphasize collaborative practice among doctors, nurses, and allied health professionals, with nurses expected to actively advocate for their patients.

# Chapter 12: Dealing with Possible Microaggressions and Discrimination as a New Nurse Moving to the USA

Foreign-trained nurses may sometimes face microaggressions and discrimination as they adjust to working in the U.S. healthcare system. These experiences can be subtle or overt and may affect their confidence and sense of belonging. Common issues include:

1. **Language and Accent Bias**

- Nurses may experience comments about their accent, communication style, or assumptions about their ability to understand English.
- This can lead to unfair perceptions of being less competent, even when they are clinically skilled.

2. **Cultural Stereotyping**

- Foreign-trained nurses may encounter stereotypes about their country of origin, culture, or education.
- Colleagues or patients may make insensitive jokes or remarks that undermine their professionalism.

3. **Exclusion or Isolation**

- Some nurses may feel left out of team discussions, social activities, or professional opportunities because they are perceived as "different."

4. **Unequal Opportunities**

- They may be overlooked for promotions, leadership roles, or advanced practice positions due to bias, even when fully qualified.

5. **Patient Bias**

- Patients may occasionally request "American nurses" or express discomfort with a nurse's accent or cultural background, which can be disheartening.

6. **Microaggressions in Everyday Interactions**

   Examples include:

- "Where are you really from?"
- Being constantly asked to repeat oneself.
- Expressions of surprise when they demonstrate advanced knowledge or skills.

**Impact**

These experiences can lead to stress, job dissatisfaction, and even burnout if left unaddressed.

**Coping Strategies**

- Seek mentorship from supportive colleagues.
- Use hospital diversity, equity, and inclusion (DEI) resources.
- Build peer support networks with other international nurses.
- Advocate for cultural competence training in the workplace.

# Chapter 13: Imposter Syndrome

Imposter syndrome is very common among foreign-trained nurses entering the U.S. healthcare system. It can appear as feelings of self-doubt, fear of being "found out," or anxiety about whether you are competent enough despite your education and experience. Let's break this down into detailed guidance and strategies.

**Understanding Imposter Syndrome and Why It Happens**

1. **New environment and expectations:** U.S. healthcare systems may operate differently than those in your home country (e.g., electronic health records, protocols, legal responsibilities).
2. **Cultural adjustments:** Communication styles, teamwork, and patient interactions may feel unfamiliar.
3. **High standards and scrutiny:** You may feel pressure to prove yourself in a new professional culture.
4. **Internal comparison:** Comparing yourself to nurses trained in the U.S. can amplify self-doubt.

**Practical Strategies to Overcome It**

1. **Validate Your Competence**

- Remember that your international education and experience are valuable.
- Keep a "competency journal" where you note achievements, positive patient outcomes, or skills mastered.

- Celebrate small wins daily.

2. **Seek Mentorship**

- Identify experienced nurses, ideally someone who understands the challenges of foreign-trained professionals.
- Mentors can provide guidance, reassurance, and practical tips for navigating the U.S. system.

3. **Prepare and Learn Continuously**

- Attend hospital orientation programs thoroughly.
- Take advantage of online courses (e.g., ICU basics, patient safety, or EHR training).
- Understand state-specific nursing laws and scope of practice.

4. **Develop a Support Network**

- Join professional associations (e.g., the American Nurses Association or the International Nurses Society).
- Connect with other foreign-trained nurses to share experiences and coping strategies.

5. **Reframe Negative Thoughts**

- Replace thoughts like "I don't belong here" with "I am learning and growing."
- Recognize that learning curves are normal for everyone, even U.S.-trained nurses.

6. **Practice Self-Compassion**

- Give yourself permission to make mistakes—they are learning opportunities.
- Use mindfulness, journaling, or stress-management techniques to reduce anxiety.

7. **Focus on Evidence-Based Confidence**

- Remind yourself of your qualifications: NCLEX pass, visa approval, clinical experience.
- Keep track of patient feedback, preceptor evaluations, and certifications earned.

8. **Set Realistic Goals**

- Break tasks into small steps, such as mastering EHR documentation before tackling complex patient assessments.
- Recognize progress rather than expecting instant perfection.

**Extra Tips for Foreign-Trained Nurses**

- **Understand U.S. jargon:** Medical terminology, abbreviations, and documentation styles may differ from those in your home country.
- **Ask questions:** Asking shows diligence, not incompetence.
- **Observe before acting:** Watch how colleagues interact, then gradually integrate your own style.

- **Learn hospital culture:** Each institution has its own workflow, hierarchy, and communication norms.

### When to Seek Extra Help

- Persistent anxiety or self-doubt that affects your work or personal life.
- Feelings of depression or burnout.
- If necessary, consider speaking with a counselor or psychologist who specializes in workplace stress for healthcare professionals.

### Key Mindset Shift

Imposter syndrome doesn't mean you are not capable—it means you are challenging yourself and growing. Every foreign-trained nurse has to navigate the learning curve, and your success depends on persistence, continuous learning, and strong support networks.

# CONFIDENCE ROADMAP

6-month plan for reducing imposter syndrome and building confidence as a foreign-trained nurse in the U.

## MONTH 1

### ORIENTATION & OBSERVATION

Understand your new environment and identify learning gaps →

Actions: Attend all hospital orientation sessions thoroughly (policies: EMR/EHR systems, safety protocols)

Shadow experienced hurses to observe workfiaw, patient interrction, and documentation style

Keep a journal of daily challenges and successes, no motter how smail

Tips: Don't hesitate to ask questions– curiosity is a strength, not a weakness.

## MONTH 2

### SKILL ASSESSMENT & CONFIDENCE BUILDING

identify areas where extra practice or learning lo nee-ded

Actions: List all nursing skills you teal less confident about and practice them under-supervision

Attend optional workshops or online courses (e.g. IV insertion, EHR training, patient safety)

Ask your mentor or preceptor for feedback and constructive guida-

Start reframing negative thoughts into learning statements (e.g. "I'm learning this new system; it's okay not to know everything yet')

## MONTH 3

### NETWORK & MENTORSHIP

Build a professional support system ←

Actions: Join local or national nursing associations (e.g., A'NA, international Nurses Society)

Find a mentor– ideally someone familiar with foreign-trained nurse challenges

Connect with peets who have successfully transitioned to U.S. nursing

Attend informal social or professional events to bulld relationships

## MONTH 4

### DEEPEN CLINICAL KNOWLEDGE

Strengthen confidence in patient care and clinical desision-making

Actions: Focus on evidence-based practice: review unit-specific protocols and procedures

Begin mentoring newer foreign-trained nurses if possible– it reinforces your own khowledge

Seek feedback regularly to continue improving performance

Practice assertive communication with colleagues and patients

**Tip:** Realize that confidence of-

# Chapter 14: Academic Growth

This chapter focuses on continuing education: obtaining your BSN, selecting a school, weighing the pros and cons of online programs, choosing a career path, deciding on a degree plan, and determining payment methods or opportunities for funding.

Take some personal time to reflect. If possible, journal or create a timeline and plan for what you want your career or professional path to look like in the near future. This will help guide you in identifying the academic steps you need to take. Acting without a plan can lead to poor time management, wasted time due to uncertainty, wasted money pursuing goals you are unsure you truly want, and delays in achieving your dream. Creating a clear plan will allow you to live out that dream to the fullest in a timely manner.

- Find a path or specialty that you love, and focus on it.
- Do as much research as you can. Don't just take my word, or anyone else's, but read and edify yourself personally.
- Capitalize on every opportunity for professional and personal growth. This will help you learn to work more efficiently and effectively.
- If possible, avoid student loans. Explore options such as paying out of pocket, scholarships, and educational grants to help subsidize costs. If student loans are your only alternative, make

sure you have a solid repayment plan so you don't end up bankrupt in the long run.

- Life is a balance. Try to strike a healthy balance between work, school, family life, and personal time. Make room to renew your energy and have fun; otherwise, you risk burnout.
- Take a break if needed, but don't give up. If you feel worn out by a busy schedule, don't make rash decisions. Step back, reassess your situation, and then move forward. As the famous quote says: *"When you feel like quitting, think of why you started."*
- Shop around for schools. Many institutions will tell you what you want to hear, but after enrollment you may find a different reality. Reading and research are key. Keep your options open, compare tuition fees, explore scholarships, review program durations, read online reviews, and seek advice from your employer's education department.
- My BSN program at GCU took 16 months to complete. During that time, I made the President's List twice, was accepted into two prestigious honor societies (Sigma Theta Tau and NCSC), and graduated with a 3.83 GPA, earning Cum Laude and University Honors. Afterward, I took a one-month break to rest—long enough to recharge but not so long that I lost my study rhythm. I then began my Master's in Nursing with an emphasis on leadership in the healthcare system.

**Online vs in-person nursing education. Pros and cons. Let's break it down for you.**

Here's a detailed comparison of online nursing education versus in-person nursing education, with pros and cons for each. I'll break it down into key factors:

1. **Learning Environment**

*Online Nursing Education Pros:*

- Flexible schedule—can study from anywhere, which is great if you're working or have family responsibilities.
- Self-paced learning is often possible, letting you spend more time on difficult topics.

*Cons:*

- Less hands-on experience in person; clinical skills may be harder to master without physical practice.
- Fewer opportunities for spontaneous interaction with instructors or peers.

*In-Person Nursing Education Pros:*

- Direct access to instructors for immediate questions and feedback.
- Hands-on labs and clinical simulations help reinforce skills.
- Stronger peer support and networking opportunities.

*Cons:*

- Less flexibility—set class schedules and commuting time.
- Harder to balance with work or family obligations.

2. **Clinical Experience Online**

- Many programs require in-person clinical rotations locally, which can limit options.
- Simulated labs online may not fully replicate real patient care.

*In-Person*

- Integrated clinical rotations and skills labs give practical experience with patients, equipment, and procedures.
- Easier to build confidence in real-life nursing situations.

3. **Cost and Resources**

*Online Pros:*

- Often cheaper; no commuting or relocation costs.
- Digital resources are readily available.

*Cons:*

- May require a strong home study environment and reliable internet.

*In-Person Pros:*

- Full access to campus resources (labs, libraries, support services).

*Cons:*

- Tuition can be higher; commuting and housing costs may add up.

4. **Networking and Career Opportunities**

*Online*

- Networking is possible but mostly virtual—less chance for in-person mentorship.
- Some employers prefer graduates from traditional programs with in-person experience.

*In-Person*

- Stronger professional connections through clinical rotations, campus events, and instructors.
- Easier to get letters of recommendation or job referrals.

5. **Learning Style Compatibility Online**

- Ideal for self-motivated, independent learners who thrive on digital resources.
- Can be challenging for those who learn best through hands-on practice or face-to-face instruction.

*In-Person*

- Suits learners who benefit from structured schedules, direct feedback, and interactive environments.

- Less flexible for nontraditional students or those balancing multiple responsibilities.

**Summary Table**

| **Factor** | **Online Nursing** | **In-Person Nursing** |
|---|---|---|
| Flexibility | High | Low |
| Hands-on skills | Limited | Excellent |
| Networking | Mostly virtual | Strong |
| Cost | Often lower | Often higher |
| Learning style | Self-motivated | Structured, guided |
| Career readiness | May need extra clinical practice | Direct exposure to real-world nursing |

**Key Insight:**

Many modern programs combine online coursework with local clinical rotations— giving flexibility without sacrificing hands-on experience. If you need convenience and self-paced study, online is great. If you prioritize hands-on skills, mentorship, and networking, in-person may be better.

# Chapter 15: Payment Opportunities for Nursing Program (Grants, Scholarships, Loans, etc.)

If you're a foreign-educated nurse planning to study in the U.S., or a nurse already in the U.S. seeking financial assistance for nursing programs (ADN, BSN, MSN), there are several avenues to explore. Here's a comprehensive guide to help you navigate funding options:

**Financial Aid Options for Nursing Programs**

1. **University-Specific Scholarships and Grants**

Many U.S. nursing schools offer scholarships and grants to international students:

- **Johns Hopkins School of Nursing:** International students are automatically considered for merit-based scholarships; however, need-based financial aid is reserved for U.S. citizens and permanent residents.
- **Yale School of Nursing:** International applicants may be considered for need-based funding by submitting a YSN financial aid form.
- **University of Washington School of Nursing:** Offers various funding opportunities for nursing students, both within the School of Nursing and the broader university community.

- **University of San Francisco School of Nursing:** Requires international students to provide proof of funds, such as bank statements or sponsor letters, to cover tuition and living expenses.
- **Chamberlain University:** Awarded more than $81 million in scholarships and grants in 2024, offering various financial aid options for nursing students.

2. **External Scholarships and Grants**

Several organizations provide scholarships and grants to nursing students:

- **BridgeWay Nursing Scholarship:** Offers fully funded scholarships for international students pursuing master's degrees in high-demand nursing specializations.
- **American Nephrology Nurses' Association (ANNA):** Provides scholarship opportunities for members working on a BSN or advanced nursing degree.
- **NurseJournal.org:** Lists various scholarships for international nursing students pursuing ADN, BSN, or MSN programs.

3. **Loan Forgiveness and Repayment Programs**

While international students may not qualify for U.S. federal student loans, other funding options are available:

- **Nurse Corps Scholarship Program:** Covers tuition, fees, and other educational costs, along with a monthly stipend, in exchange for working at a health care facility with a critical shortage of nurses after graduation.

- **National Health Service Corps (NHSC):** Provides loan repayment assistance for nurses working in underserved areas.

4. **Private Loans and Funding**

International students may also explore private loan options to finance their education:

- **Private Student Loans:** Some U.S. lenders offer private loans to international students, often requiring a creditworthy U.S. co-signer.
- **Home Country Scholarships:** Check with your home country's government or educational agencies for potential scholarships or loan programs to support study abroad.

**Application Tips**

- **Prepare Financial Documentation:** Be ready to provide proof of funds, such as bank statements or sponsor letters, to demonstrate your ability to cover tuition and living expenses.
- **Meet Deadlines:** Adhere to application deadlines for scholarships, grants, and admissions to ensure full consideration.
- **Seek Guidance:** Utilize resources like EducationUSA for advice on U.S. higher education and financing options.

By exploring these resources and planning ahead, you can secure financial support to pursue your nursing education in the United States. If you need assistance with specific applications or have further questions, feel free to ask!

**U.S. Military and Nursing Education Funding**

The U.S. military provides multiple education funding benefits for nurses—covering ADN, BSN, MSN, and advanced practice programs. These benefits extend to active-duty service members, reservists, National Guard members, spouses, and dependents.

**1. Active-Duty Service Members**

**Tuition Assistance (TA)**

- **Who:** Active-duty personnel (all branches)
- **Coverage:** Up to 100% tuition; typically, $250 per semester credit hour or $4,500 per fiscal year
- **Eligibility:** Must be on active duty with command approval
- **Use:** Undergraduate (ADN/BSN) and graduate (MSN) nursing programs

**GI Bill / Post-9/11 GI Bill**

- **Who:** Veterans with at least 90 days of active duty since 9/11
- **Coverage:** Tuition, fees, housing, books, and supplies
- **Use:** BSN, MSN, and doctoral programs (including online)

- **Extras:** Some branches offer Top-Up programs if tuition exceeds GI Bill limits

**Health Professions Scholarship Program (HPSP)**

- **Who:** Nursing and other health profession students entering service
- **Coverage:** Full tuition + monthly stipend (~$2,000) + health insurance
- **Commitment:** 2–4 years of active duty after graduation

**2. Reserve and National Guard Members**

**Tuition Assistance**

- Many Reserve and Guard units offer tuition aid similar to active duty, though amounts may vary by state.

**Montgomery GI Bill – Selected Reserve (MGIB-SR)**

- **Who:** Reserve and Guard members
- **Coverage:** Monthly stipend for tuition and fees
- **Notes:** Can be combined with federal grants

**State Tuition Assistance Programs**

- Many states offer additional in-state tuition support for Guard members, covering partial or full tuition.

**3. Spouses and Family Members**

**MyCAA – Military Spouse Career Advancement Accounts**

- **Who:** Spouses of active-duty and certain Reserve members

- **Coverage:** Up to $4,000 for tuition, fees, certifications, or licensing
- **Eligibility:** For associate or bachelor's programs in portable careers (nursing included)
- **Use:** ADN, BSN, RN-to-BSN programs

**Post-9/11 GI Bill Transfer**

- **Who:** Service members with at least 6 years of service
- **Coverage:** Transfer unused GI Bill benefits to spouses or children
- **Use:** Full tuition + housing allowance for nursing education

**4. Additional Support Programs**

- **Loan Repayment Programs:** Available in high-need specialties or hard-to-fill areas
- **Branch-Specific Scholarships:** e.g., Army Nurse Corps, Navy Nurse Corps

**Key Tips**

1. **Combine Benefits:** Tuition assistance, GI Bill, and scholarships can be used together to maximize funding.
2. **Plan Early:** Programs like HPSP require early application.
3. **Check State Options:** National Guard members often qualify for state-based tuition reimbursement.

4. **Consider Online Programs:** Many military benefits cover accredited online nursing programs for flexibility.

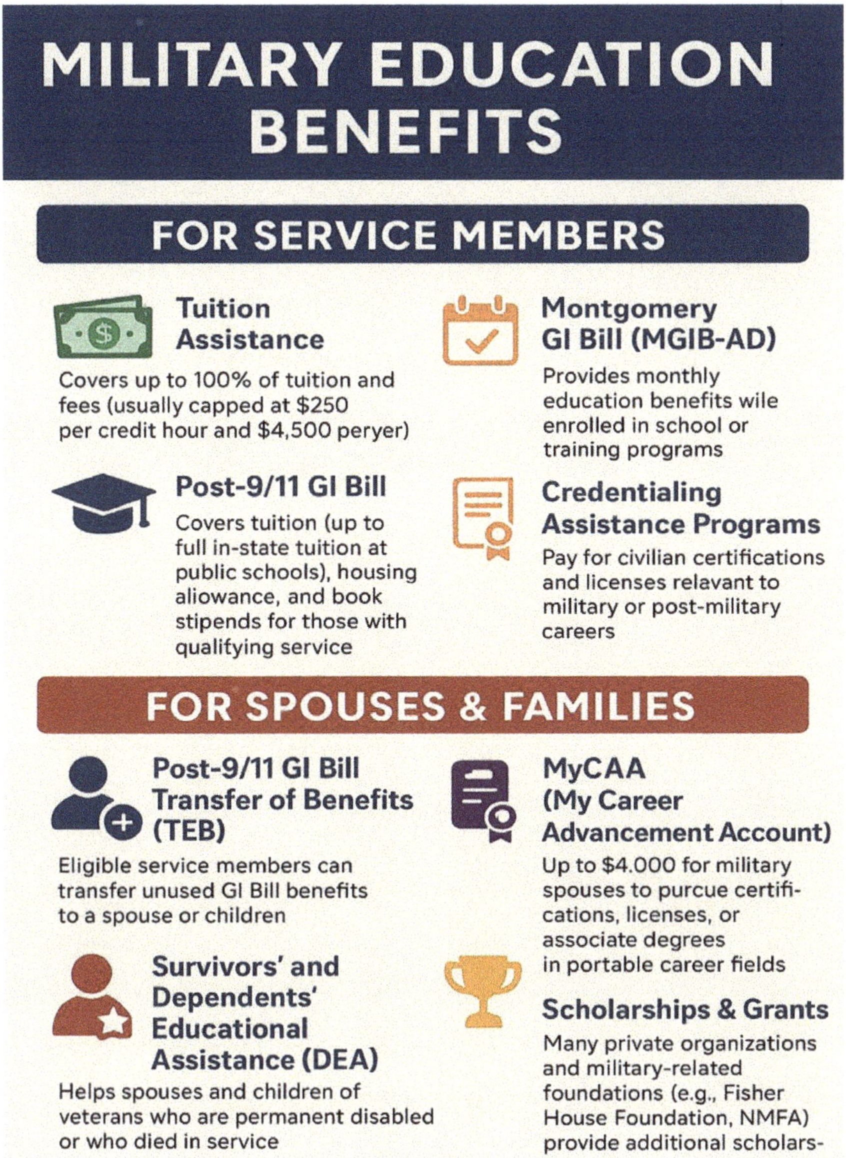

# Chapter 16: How Did I Personally Pay for My Bachelor's and Master's Degrees Without Taking School Loans or Being in Debt?

When I came to the USA, I knew I wanted to go back to school, but I had to figure out how to do so without incurring debt or taking student loans. I met an unreal number of people—many of them nurses—who, after completing their degrees, were struggling to repay student loans or dealing with significant credit card debt. I knew this was something I did not want to face.

So, I did some research, which led me to two options that worked for me. For my Bachelor's degree, I was working full-time, so I checked to see if I qualified for any student aid through Studentaid.gov, a government website and app where you can apply for and determine eligibility for grants, loans, and scholarships. I was specifically looking for aid I would not need to repay. This led me to a Pell Grant. So, what is a Pell Grant?

*"Federal Pell Grants usually are awarded only to undergraduate students who display exceptional financial need and have not earned a bachelor's, graduate, or professional degree."*

studentaid.gov/understand-aid/types/grants/pell

You do not need to repay Pell Grants once you qualify—they are grants, not loans. You will be asked a series of questions and required to submit documents such as tax information, employment details, and household income, among other items. Then, you will receive feedback on whether you qualify for a Pell Grant and how much you are eligible for.

*"The amount you get, though, will depend on your Student Aid Index (based on your FAFSA form), the cost of attendance (determined by your school for your specific program), your status as a full-time or part-time student, and your plans to attend school for a full academic year or less."*

studentaid.gov/understand-aid/types/grants/pell#how-apply

For me, the Pell Grant covered a little more than half of my Bachelor's program, which was significant. Since I was working, I paid the remaining balance out of pocket per course. This provided tremendous financial relief.

For my Master's degree, I took a different route. I was looking for funding that covered the entire program without out-of-pocket costs. At the time, my husband was serving in the U.S. military as a Marine and received educational benefits, including the GI Bill. This program allows active-duty personnel to either pay for school fully or transfer all or part of the benefit to their spouse or children. I utilized part of his GI Bill benefit to cover my entire Master's degree—without paying anything out of pocket. I am deeply thankful for this opportunity afforded by the federal government to military families.

I am now using similar methods to cover the cost of my Nurse Practitioner program.

# Chapter 17: Hospitals/ Jobs Funding Nursing Education Programs and Offering Loan Forgiveness

Many hospitals in the U.S. offer programs to help nurses pay for further education, ranging from ADN → BSN, BSN → MSN, or advanced practice programs. Here's a detailed overview of how hospital-funded nursing education typically works:

**1. Tuition Reimbursement / Tuition Assistance Programs**

- **What it is:** Hospitals pay all or part of your tuition for approved nursing programs.
- **Eligibility:** Often requires full-time or part-time employment, sometimes after a minimum tenure (e.g., 6–12 months).
- **Requirements:** Maintain a certain GPA and continue working at the hospital for a specified time after completion.
- **Coverage:** Can range from a few thousand dollars per year to full tuition coverage; some programs also cover books and fees.
- **Examples of hospitals offering this:**
  - **Mayo Clinic:** Tuition reimbursement for BSN and higher degrees.
  - **Cleveland Clinic:** Tuition reimbursement for nursing and allied health programs.

- **Johns Hopkins Hospital:** Tuition assistance and loan repayment programs.

**2. Loan Forgiveness or Repayment Programs**

- **What it is:** Hospitals may pay off a portion of student loans in exchange for a set number of years of service.
- **How it works:** Often targeted at nurses with BSN, MSN, or advanced practice degrees.
- **Benefits:** Can be combined with federal programs such as Public Service Loan Forgiveness (PSLF).

**3. Scholarship Programs**

- Some hospitals offer internal scholarships specifically for nurses continuing their education.
- **Eligibility:** Usually merit- or need-based, sometimes focused on underserved specialties (e.g., ICU, ER, OR).
- **Amount:** Ranges from $1,000–$5,000+ per year, sometimes renewable.

**4. Flexible Scheduling / Paid Study Leave**

Even if tuition isn't fully covered, hospitals may provide:

- Flexible shifts to attend classes.
- Paid study leaves for exams or clinical rotations.
- Coverage for continuing education units (CEUs) required for licensure.

**5. Types of Programs Supported**

- **ADN → BSN:** Very common; hospitals often encourage RNs to earn BSNs.
- **BSN → MSN or NP programs:** Frequently supported at teaching hospitals or Magnet-recognized hospitals.
- **Specialty certifications:** Some hospitals cover costs for certifications such as CCRN, CNOR, or CEN.

**6. Considerations Before Applying**

- **Service commitment:** Many programs require a 1–3 year work commitment after graduation.
- **Eligibility criteria:** Minimum GPA or specific work history may be required.
- **Reimbursement limits:** Some hospitals cap the amount per year or per degree.
- **Approved schools:** Benefits are often limited to accredited programs.

**7. How to Find Out What's Available**

- Check with your hospital's HR or Education Department.
- Search for "tuition reimbursement" or "nursing education assistance" in the employee handbook or intranet.
- Ask fellow nurses; they often know which programs are most accessible.

# Chapter 18: How Should Foreign-Educated Nurses Select Schools for Educational Advancement for BSN, MSN or Advanced Practice Programs?

When a foreign-educated nurse is considering further education in the U.S.—whether a BSN, MSN, or advanced practice (NP, CNS, CRNA, CNM) program—careful selection of the school is crucial. Here's a structured approach to make the decision strategically:

1. **Accreditation and Recognition**

   Check the accrediting bodies:

- BSN/MSN: Look for CCNE (Commission on Collegiate Nursing Education) or ACEN (Accreditation Commission for Education in Nursing) accreditation.
- Advanced practice programs: Ensure the program meets the APRN (Advanced Practice Registered Nurse) competencies recognized by AANP or NONPF.
- Accreditation affects licensure eligibility, eligibility for federal financial aid, and employment opportunities.

2. **State Licensure Alignment**

- Verify the school's curriculum aligns with the state board of nursing requirements where you plan to practice.

- Some states have specific clinical hour requirements or coursework for advanced practice licensure.

3. **Program Type and Pathways for Foreign-Educated Nurses**

- RN-to-BSN programs: Designed for nurses with a diploma or associate degree; many accept international RN credentials after U.S. licensure.
- Direct-entry MSN programs: If you have a non-nursing bachelor's degree but want an advanced practice career.
- Bridge programs: Some universities offer accelerated BSN or foreign-educated nurse programs, helping meet U.S. academic standards efficiently.

4. **Clinical Placement Opportunities**

- Check if the school has strong partnerships with hospitals and clinics for clinical rotations, especially for advanced practice students.
- The quality and variety of clinical experiences directly impact learning and licensure preparedness.

5. **International Student Support**

Look for programs with:

- ESL or academic writing support
- Visa/immigration advising
- Cultural orientation for healthcare practice in the U.S.
- Programs tailored to foreign-educated nurses may also help navigate U.S. healthcare systems and expectations.

6. **Flexibility and Delivery Mode**

- Online vs. in-person: Some schools offer hybrid or fully online programs, which may help working nurses.
- Accelerated options: If you want to fast-track career advancement, check for accelerated BSN or MSN tracks.

7. **Outcomes and Reputation Review**

- NCLEX pass rates (for BSN programs if you are obtaining U.S. RN licensure)
- Certification exam passes rates (for MSN/APRN programs)
- Graduate employment statistics
- Check school rankings and feedback from foreign-educated nurse alumni.

8. **Financial Considerations**

- Tuition and fees vary widely; also factor in living expenses.
- Explore scholarships, assistantships, or grants available for international nurses.

9. **Specialty Options**

- If you aim for advanced practice, ensure the school offers your desired specialty (e.g., family NP, pediatric NP, nurse anesthetist).
- Some programs are limited in clinical specialties or geographic locations for placements.

**10. Networking and Professional Development**

Consider schools with active nursing organizations, mentorship programs, and research opportunities, which can help you integrate into U.S. professional circles.

**Summary Recommendation:**

Foreign-educated nurses should prioritize accreditation, state licensure alignment, clinical opportunities, and program support for international students, while balancing specialty interests, flexibility, and financial feasibility. Visiting campuses, talking to program directors, and connecting with alumni can provide practical insights that online research might miss.

Here's a step-by-step checklist tailored for foreign-educated nurses to evaluate BSN, MSN, and advanced practice programs in the U.S.:

**Step-by-Step School Selection Checklist for Foreign-Educated Nurses**

***Step 1: Verify Accreditation***

- Is the program CCNE or ACEN accredited?
- For advanced practice: Does it meet AANP/NONPF standards for your specialty?
- Will the degree qualify you for U.S. licensure exams (NCLEX for BSN, certification for APRN)?

***Step 2: Confirm State Licensure Compatibility***

- Is the program recognized by the State Board of Nursing where you want to practice?
- Does it meet clinical hour requirements and coursework expectations for licensure?
- If you are in a compact state, check multistate license acceptance.

***Step 3: Check Program Type and Pathway***

- Is this program suited for your current nursing background?
- RN diploma → RN-to-BSN
- Non-nursing bachelor's → Direct-entry MSN
- Foreign RN → Bridge programs or accelerated tracks
- Does it allow you to transfer credits from previous education?

***Step 4: Evaluate Clinical Opportunities***

- Does the school provide diverse clinical rotations aligned with your specialty?
- Are preceptors experienced in working with international students?
- Is there flexibility in clinical sites or location options?

***Step 5: Assess Support for International Students***

- Does the school provide ESL support, academic writing help, or tutoring?
- Is there visa and immigration guidance?

- Are there cultural orientation programs for U.S. healthcare settings?

***Step 6: Determine Delivery Mode & Flexibility***

- Is the program in-person, online, or hybrid?
- Are there accelerated or part-time options for working nurses?
- Does the program allow practical experience locally if online?

***Step 7: Review Outcomes and Reputation***

- NCLEX pass rate (for BSN programs)
- Specialty certification passes rate (for MSN/APRN)
- Graduate employment rate & types of employers
- Alumni network and mentoring opportunities

***Step 8: Financial Considerations***

- Tuition, fees, and estimated living costs
- Availability of scholarships, grants, or assistantships for international students
- Cost-benefit analysis: program prestige vs. debt vs. career outcome

***Step 9: Confirm Specialty Options***

- Does the school offer your desired advanced practice specialty?
- Are there adequate clinical placements for that specialty?
- Are research, leadership, or elective courses relevant to your goals available?

***Step 10: Professional Networking Opportunities***

- Does the program offer student nursing organizations or professional mentorship?
- Are there research, conference, or clinical networking opportunities?
- Can the school connect you with alumni working in U.S. healthcare?

# Chapter 19: Nursing Certification and Specialization, Why Should I Become Certified or Specialized?

Choosing a nursing specialty and pursuing certifications is a crucial step in shaping your career. Let's break it down into clear steps and considerations:

**1. Understanding Nursing Certifications**

***Definition:***

Nursing certifications are credentials that validate your expertise in a specific area of practice beyond your basic RN license. They show employers and patients that you have advanced knowledge and skills in a specialty.

***Types of Certifications:***

1. Entry-level Certifications: For newly licensed nurses looking to specialize.

Example: Certified Pediatric Nurse (CPN) for nurses in pediatrics.

2. Advanced Certifications: For experienced nurses seeking leadership, education, or clinical mastery.

Example: Critical Care Registered Nurse (CCRN) or Family Nurse Practitioner (FNP).

***Benefits of Certification:***

- Demonstrates advanced competency in a specialty.
- Can lead to higher salary or promotion opportunities.
- Increases job security and professional credibility.
- Sometimes required for certain roles or hospital units.

***How to Get Certified:***

1. Meet eligibility requirements (usually a combination of RN license + clinical hours in the specialty).

2. Complete required continuing education or specialty training.

3. Pass the specialty certification exam.

4. Maintain certification through periodic renewal, which may involve continuing education or re-examination.

***Resources for Certification Info:***

- American Nurses Credentialing Center (ANCC)
- American Association of Critical-Care Nurses (AACN)
- Specialty Nursing Organizations (e.g., Pediatric Nursing Certification Board, Oncology Nursing Society)

**2. Choosing a Nursing Specialty**

***Factors to Consider:***

1. Personal Interests and Passion:

- Think about the patient populations you enjoy working with (children, adults, elderly).

- Consider the type of care environment you prefer (ICU, outpatient, community health).

2. Work-Life Balance:

- Some specialties have more predictable schedules (e.g., outpatient, school nursing).
- Others like ER, ICU, or labor & delivery may involve night shifts and high-stress environments.

3. Salary Potential:

- Specialty certifications often lead to higher pay.
- Examples: CRNA (nurse anesthetist) and NP roles usually pay more than general med-surg nursing.

4. Long-Term Career Goals:

- Do you want to move into advanced practice, management, or education?
- Some specialties are stepping stones for higher roles.

5. Job Market Demand:

- Research which specialties are in high demand in your region.
- High-demand areas often provide more job security and benefits.

**Popular Nursing Specialties:**

- Critical Care (ICU), Hospital ICU, CCRN (critical care registered nurse) High-stress, high pay

- Emergency Nursing, ER. CEN (Certified Emergency Nurse) Fast-paced, acute care
- Pediatric- Children's hospitals, clinic, CPN (certified pediatric nurse) Focus on children's health
- Oncology- Cancer centers, hospitals, OCN (Oncology Certified Nurse) Emotional, rewarding
- Labor & Delivery- Hospitals. RNC-LRN. Focus on childbirth
- Psychiatric / Mental Health- Mental health facilities. PMH-BC (Psychiatric mental health) Growing demand
- Nurse Practitioner (NP)-Clinics, hospitals. FNP (family nurse practitioner), AGACNP (adult- gerontology Acute care nurse), PNP (psychiatric nurse practitioner). Advanced practice with autonomy
- Geriatrics- Nursing homes, home health. GNP-BC (Geriatric nurse practitioner), Growing with aging population
- Informatics / Education- Hospitals, schools. RN-BC (board certified nurse educator or nurse informatics) non-clinical, tech & teaching roles

**3. Steps to Decide Your Specialty:**

***1. Self-Assessment:***

Identify your strengths, interests, and preferred work environment.

***2. Research:***

Look into roles, certifications, salary, and job outlook.

***3. Shadow / Volunteer:***

Gain firsthand experience in different units or specialties.

***4. Talk to Mentors:***

Ask experienced nurses about their day-to-day work and satisfaction.

***5. Start General, Then Specialize:***

Many nurses begin in Med-Surg or ICU, then move into a specialty as they gain experience.

***6. Plan for Certification:***

Once you pick a specialty, check which certifications are most respected and align with your career goals.

# Chapter 20: Understanding Health Insurance, Taxes, Credit Score and Retirement Plan as a Foreign-Educated Nurse Transitioning to the USA

These four topics are crucial for a smooth financial and personal transition but can feel overwhelming for foreign-educated nurses coming to the U.S. Here's a clear, nurse-friendly breakdown:

**Health Insurance**

Employer-based coverage: Most hospitals and clinics provide health insurance. The cost is usually shared between the employer and the employee.

***Key Terms to Know:***

- Premium: what you pay monthly for insurance.
- Deductible: what you pay out-of-pocket before insurance starts covering costs.
- Copay: fixed amount you pay for a doctor visit, ER, or medication.
- Out-of-pocket maximum: the highest you'll pay in a year; after that, insurance covers 100%.
- Tip for new nurses: Always choose a plan that includes your local hospitals and clinics (in-network providers).

**Taxes**

- **Federal income tax:** Paid to the U.S. government; depends on income bracket.
- **State income tax:** Some states (like Texas, Florida, and Nevada) have no state income tax; others do.
- **Payroll deductions:** Medicare and Social Security are automatically taken from your paycheck.
- **Tax filing:** Every April, you must file taxes (Form 1040). Many nurses use TurboTax, H&R Block, or an accountant.
- **Tip for new nurses:** Keep pay stubs and W-2 forms; you may qualify for deductions (education, moving expenses in some cases).

**Credit Score**

A credit score (300–850) shows how financially trustworthy you are.

Why it matters: Affects your ability to rent an apartment, buy a car/house, or even get loans.

***How to build credit:***

1. Open a U.S. bank account and get a secured credit card.
2. Pay all bills on time (rent, phone, utilities).
3. Keep credit card balances low (under 30% of the limit).

Tip for new nurses: Start small with one card; good credit takes time to build.

**Retirement Plans**

- **401(k) or 403(b):** Employer-sponsored retirement plans.
  - Hospitals (nonprofits) often use 403(b), while private companies use 401(k).
  - You can contribute a portion of your paycheck before taxes.
  - Many employers match contributions (free money!).
- **Social Security:** Nurses working legally in the U.S. pay into Social Security through payroll taxes and can claim benefits later (usually after 10 years of work).
- **Other Options:** Nurses can also open IRAs (Individual Retirement Accounts) for extra savings.

**Tip for New Nurses:** Start contributing early — even a small percentage can grow significantly over time through compound interest.

**Quick Example for a New Nurse**

- A hospital offers health insurance and a 403(b) retirement plan with a 5% match.
- You sign up, pay a small monthly premium, and contribute 5% of your paycheck.
- You pay federal and state taxes, build credit with a secured card, and by year 2–3, you're financially stable and eligible for bigger opportunities (car, homeownership, travel).

## Financial Survival Guide for Foreign-Educated Nurses in the USA

Transitioning into the U.S. healthcare system is more than just passing the NCLEX — understanding money, benefits, and financial systems is key to thriving. Here's what every nurse should know:

### Health Insurance

**Employer-Based Coverage:** Most hospitals and clinics provide insurance, with costs shared between you and your employer.

**Key Terms:**

- **Premium:** Monthly cost to have insurance.
- **Deductible:** The amount you pay out of pocket before insurance begins covering costs.
- **Copay:** A small, fixed fee for doctor visits, ER visits, or medications.
- **Out-of-Pocket Maximum:** The most you'll pay in a year for healthcare.

**Tip:** Choose an in-network plan (doctors and hospitals covered by your insurance) to avoid large bills.

### Taxes

- **Federal Income Tax:** Paid to the U.S. government; deducted from each paycheck.

- **State Income Tax:** Depends on the state (e.g., no state tax in Texas, Florida, or Nevada).
- **Payroll Deductions:** Medicare and Social Security are taken out automatically.
- **Tax Filing:** Every April, you must file a tax return (Form 1040). Keep your W-2 form from your employer.

**Tip:** Use services like TurboTax, H&R Block, or an accountant to file correctly.

**Credit Score**

**What It Is:** A number (300–850) showing how responsible you are with money.

**Why It Matters:** It's needed for renting an apartment, buying a car or house, or applying for loans.

**How to Build:**

1. Open a U.S. bank account.
2. Apply for a secured credit card.
3. Always pay bills on time.
4. Keep balances under 30% of your credit limit.

**Tip:** Building good credit takes time—start small and stay consistent.

**Retirement Plans**

- **401(k)/403(b):** Retirement savings offered by most hospitals. Pre-tax money from your paycheck goes into the plan. Employers often match part of your contribution (free money!).
- **Social Security:** You pay into this with payroll deductions and can access benefits after working about 10 years.
- **Extra Savings:** Nurses can also open an IRA (Individual Retirement Account).

**Tip:** Start contributing early, even 3–5% of your paycheck. Small amounts grow into big savings over time.

**Quick Example for a New Nurse**

- **Monthly Paycheck:** $4,500
    - $500 → Federal/State Taxes
    - $150 → Health Insurance Premium
    - $225 → Retirement Contribution (5%)
    - Employer matches $225 → Your retirement savings grow faster.

By using a secured credit card and paying bills on time, your credit score can jump to 700+ within a year.

**Key Takeaways**

- Sign up for health insurance right away.
- File your taxes on time every April.

- Start building a credit score as soon as possible.
- Don't wait to save—small retirement contributions add up.

# Financial Survival Guide

## for Foreign-Educated Nurses in the USA

Transitioning into the U.S. healthcare system is more than just passing the NCLEX— understanding money, benefits, and financial systems is key to thriving. Here's what every nurse should know.

### Health Insurance

- **Employer-Based Coverage**
- Most hospitals and clinics provide insurance. Costs are shared between you and your employer
- **Key Terms**

  **Premium** → Monthly cost to have insurance

  **Deductible** → The amount you pay out-of-pocket before insurance kicks in

  **Copay** → Small set fee for doctor visits, ER, or medication

  **Out-of-Pockct Maximum** → The most you'll pay in a year for healthcare

**Tip:** Choose an in-network plan (doctors/hospitals under your insurance) to avoid huge bills

### Credit Score

**What it Is**

A number (300–850) showing how responsible you are with money

### Taxes

- **Federal Income Tax**
  Paid to the U.S. governnment: taken from each paycheck
- **State Income Tax**
  Depends on the state (e.g., no state tax in Texas, Florida, Nevala)
- **Payroll Deductions**
  Medicare and Social Security come out automatically

**Tip:** Use services like TurboTax. H&R Block, or an accountant to file correctly

### Retirement Plans

- **401(k)/403(b)**
  Retirement savings offered by most hospitals
- **Pre-tax money** from your paycheck goes into the plan
- **Employers** often match part of your contribution (free money!)
- **Extra Savings**

# Chapter 21: Balancing Study and Work

Balancing nursing work, life, and studying can feel like juggling flaming swords challenging, but possible with strategy and discipline. Here's a thorough guide to make it manageable:

**1. Prioritize & Plan**

- **Set clear goals:** Define what you want to achieve in work, life, and study. For example: "Pass my certification exam in 3 months" or "Spend weekends with family."
- **Use a planner or digital calendar:** Schedule shifts, study sessions, self-care, and family time. Color-coding can help visualize your balance.

**2. Manage Time Wisely**

- **Break tasks into small chunks:** Study for 25–50 minutes, then take a 5–10 minute break (Pomodoro technique). This maintains focus without burnout.
- **Maximize downtime:** Use commute time or lunch breaks for quick reviews, podcasts, or flashcards.
- **Avoid multitasking:** Nursing work is demanding—focus on one task at a time for better efficiency.

**3. Set Boundaries**

- **Work-life boundaries:** Learn to say no when work demands spill into personal time. Overcommitting can lead to burnout.

- **Study boundaries:** Treat study time as non-negotiable. Inform friends or family of your schedule to minimize distractions.

**4. Take Care of Your Health**

- **Sleep:** Aim for 6–7 hours, even if it means cutting nonessential activities.
- **Exercise:** Short workouts or stretching can boost energy and reduce stress.
- **Nutrition:** Balanced meals sustain focus during long shifts and study sessions.

**5. Use Efficient Study Strategies**

- **Focus on high-yield content:** Identify key concepts or frequently tested topics.
- **Active learning:** Use practice questions, flashcards, or teach-back methods instead of passive reading.
- **Group study:** Join colleagues or online study groups for motivation and shared learning.

**6. Seek Support**

- **Mentors:** Experienced nurses can share strategies for balancing workload and study.
- **Family and friends:** Communicate your goals so they can support you.

- **Professional help:** Many institutions offer counseling or wellness programs for nurses.

**7. Accept Flexibility**

- **Understand that balance shifts:** Some weeks will lean more toward work, others toward study or family.
- **Celebrate small wins:** Completing a study module, surviving a tough shift, or taking a mental health day all count.
- **Extra tip:** Set "micro-goals" daily. Even 15–20 minutes of focused study is better than none. Consistency beats intensity in the long run.

# Chapter 22: Advice on Alternative Routes Such as Companies Hiring Foreign RN

If your goal is to work as a registered nurse (RN) in the U.S. but you are a foreign-educated nurse, there are several alternative pathways and resources beyond the traditional route of applying individually to hospitals or nursing programs. Here's a structured guide:

### 1. U.S. RN Licensure Basics

Before exploring alternative routes, you need to understand the licensure process:

- **NCLEX-RN Exam:** You must pass this to become a licensed RN in the U.S.
- **Credential Evaluation:** Organizations like CGFNS (Commission on Graduates of Foreign Nursing Schools) verify foreign credentials.
- **Visa Requirements:** Most foreign nurses work on H-1B, TN, or EB-3 visas sponsored by employers.

### 2. Agencies and Companies Hiring Foreign RNs

Several U.S. companies specialize in recruiting foreign nurses. These agencies often assist with:

- Visa sponsorship
- Credential verification
- Relocation assistance

- NCLEX prep or bridging programs

**a. Staffing & Recruitment Agencies**

- **O'Grady Peyton International** – Specializes in international nurse recruitment for U.S. hospitals.
- **Avant Healthcare Professionals** – Offers employment, visa sponsorship, and NCLEX guidance.
- **ADEX Medical Staffing** – Helps international nurses transition to U.S. licensure and employment.
- **International Recruiters of America (IRA)** – Provides relocation support and hospital placement.

**b. Hospital-Specific Programs**

Some hospitals and health systems run international nurse recruitment programs, especially in areas with nursing shortages:

- **Cleveland Clinic** – Offers international nurse programs with training and NCLEX support.
- **Mayo Clinic** – Occasionally recruits foreign nurses and provides relocation assistance.
- **HCA Healthcare** – Runs an International Nurse Program, sponsoring visas and offering orientation.

**c. U.S. Military & Public Health Programs**

- **U.S. Army, Navy, Air Force** – Hire nurses internationally in some cases; active-duty or reserve programs may provide education and licensure support.

- **Indian Health Service (IHS)** – Sometimes hires foreign-educated nurses to serve Native American communities.

**3. NCLEX Prep & Bridging Programs**

Some agencies also provide funding or preparation for the NCLEX, which is a common barrier for foreign nurses:

- **Kaplan NCLEX Review** – Widely used by hospitals recruiting international nurses.
- **Hurst Review Services** – Offers online NCLEX prep tailored for foreign RNs.
- **CGFNS Exchange Visa Program** – Combines credential evaluation with exam preparation for foreign nurses.

**4. Visa Sponsorship Notes**

Foreign nurses need employers willing to sponsor work visas:

- **H-1B Visa** – Requires a U.S. employer; less commonly used for RNs.
- **EB-3 Visa (Skilled Worker)** – The most common visa for foreign nurses; employer sponsorship required.
- **TN Visa** – Available for Canadian and Mexican nurses under USMCA.
- Some agencies also guide you through the green card process after 1–2 years of employment.

**5. Recommended Resources**

- **CGFNS International:** cgfns.org – Credential evaluation and licensure information.
- **NCSBN:** ncsbn.org – NCLEX details and state licensing information.
- **American Association of International Nurses (AAIN):** Advocacy and support network.
- **NursingJobs.com & Nurse.com:** Job boards with filters for "International RN" or "visa sponsorship."

Here's a step-by-step roadmap for foreign- educated nurses aiming to work as a U.S. RN, combining licensure, recruitment, and visa pathways:

**Step-by-Step Roadmap: Foreign Nurse → U.S. RN**

For many internationally trained nurses, working in the United States represents a chance to expand their careers, access advanced medical systems, and improve quality of life. However, the process of becoming a licensed Registered Nurse (RN) in the U.S. involves multiple steps, from credential evaluation to licensure exams, visa sponsorship, and relocation. The following roadmap breaks the journey down into clear, actionable stages.

***Step 1: Evaluate Your Credentials***

The first step is ensuring your nursing education and experience align with U.S. standards.

*Actions to take:*

1. **Submit documents to CGFNS (Commission on Graduates of Foreign Nursing Schools):** This organization verifies transcripts, licenses, and credentials to confirm eligibility. Their services are recognized by most U.S. state boards of nursing. Website: cgfns.org.
2. **Compare your nursing curriculum with U.S. requirements.** Some countries' programs differ in clinical hours or content. If gaps exist, you may need additional coursework.
3. **Demonstrate English proficiency.** Many states require exams like TOEFL or IELTS unless your nursing education was in English.

Tip: Some hospitals and agencies require CGFNS certification before offering contracts, so completing this step early is essential.

***Step 2: Choose Your Recruitment Route***

Foreign nurses generally have two main pathways: working with an agency or applying directly to hospital programs.

*Agency Recruitment*

Recruitment agencies assist with placement, visa sponsorship, NCLEX preparation, and relocation. Popular options include:

- O'Grady Peyton International
- Avant Healthcare Professionals
- ADEX Medical Staffing

- International Recruiters of America (IRA)

**Benefits:** Agencies streamline paperwork, provide exam support, and coordinate immigration—often resulting in faster placement.

**Direct Hospital Recruitment**

Some U.S. hospitals operate their own international nurse programs. Examples include:

- Cleveland Clinic International Nurse Program
- HCA Healthcare International Nurse Program
- Mayo Clinic (offers limited openings)

**Benefits:** Direct employment provides structured orientation, competitive benefits, and relocation assistance without a third-party intermediary.

***Step 3: Prepare for the NCLEX-RN Exam***

Every nurse must pass the NCLEX-RN exam to obtain licensure in the U.S. This test assesses nursing knowledge, critical thinking, and decision-making in clinical scenarios.

*Actions to take:*

- Apply for NCLEX eligibility through the state board of nursing where you intend to practice. Each state has its own requirements.

- Invest in high-quality NCLEX prep programs. Popular options include Kaplan NCLEX Review, Hurst Review Services, and UWorld (widely praised for its question bank).
- If you are working with a recruitment agency or hospital program, check whether they offer free or subsidized NCLEX preparation courses.

Passing the NCLEX is the single most important milestone for licensure, so dedicate consistent study time to this step.

***Step 4: Secure Visa Sponsorship***

To legally work in the United States, foreign nurses need an appropriate visa. The most common pathway is employer sponsorship.

*Visa options include:*

- **EB-3 Visa (Skilled Worker):** The standard route for foreign nurses; requires an employer sponsor.
- **H-1B Visa:** Rarely used for general RNs but sometimes applicable to advanced or specialized nursing roles.
- **TN Visa:** Available exclusively to Canadian and Mexican nurses under the USMCA agreement.
- **Green Card:** Many employers transition nurses to permanent residency after one to two years of employment.

*Actions to take:*

- Work closely with your agency or hospital's immigration team.

- Prepare all documentation, including passport, nursing license, credential evaluation, and proof of professional experience.
- Attend a visa interview if applying from outside the U.S.

***Step 5: Relocate and Complete Orientation***

Once your visa is approved, the next step is transitioning into the U.S. healthcare environment.

*Actions to take:*

- Participate in hospital orientation programs for foreign nurses. These sessions often cover U.S. clinical protocols, charting systems, and workplace expectations.
- Learn documentation standards and electronic health record (EHR) systems, which may differ from those abroad.
- Adapt to cultural differences in patient care, teamwork, and communication styles.

Tip: Networking with other international nurses can make relocation smoother by helping with housing, transportation, and local integration.

***Step 6: Advance Your Career***

Once you've settled into your role, think long-term about career growth.

*Options for advancement include:*

- **Further education:** Earning a BSN, MSN, or specialty certification can open doors to leadership roles or advanced practice nursing.
- **Travel nursing:** Agencies such as Aya Healthcare, Medical Solutions, and Cross Country Nurses offer opportunities for higher pay, flexible contracts, and diverse clinical experiences.
- **Professional associations:** Joining organizations like the American Nurses Association (ANA) or specialty-focused groups (ICU, ER, pediatrics, oncology, etc.) enhances networking, continuing education, and career visibility.

**Final Thoughts**

The journey from being a foreign-educated nurse to becoming a licensed U.S. RN is complex but entirely achievable with the right roadmap. From credential evaluation and NCLEX preparation to securing sponsorship and adapting to a new healthcare system, each step brings you closer to fulfilling your career aspirations. With determination, careful planning, and the support of agencies or hospital programs, international nurses can build successful and rewarding careers in the United States.

### Visual Summary: Roadmap Flow

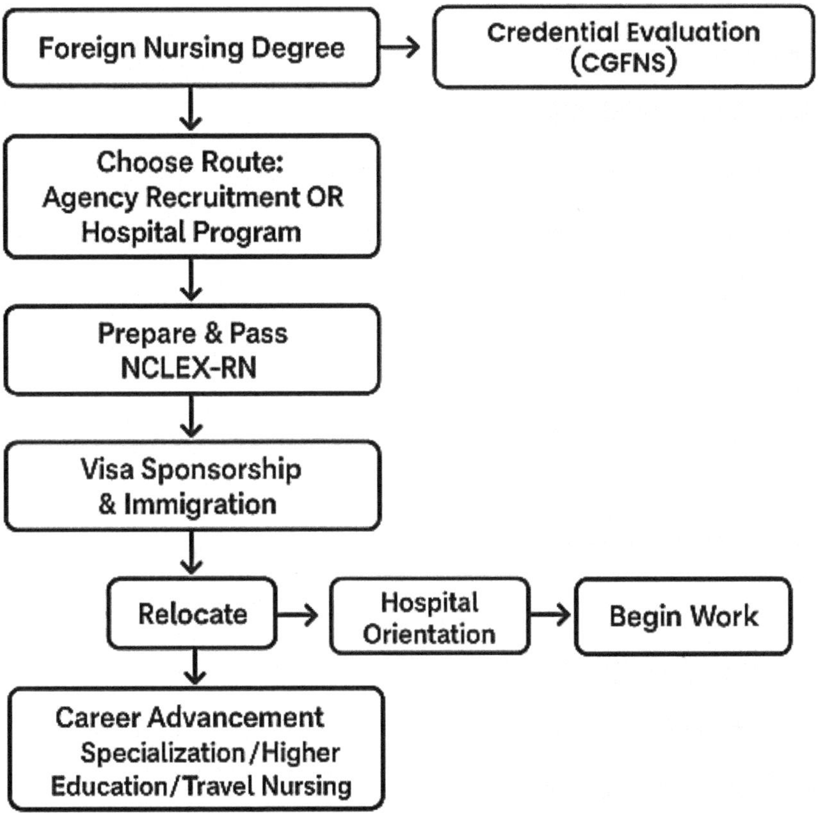

# Chapter 23: Your Journey Forward – Thriving as a Nurse in the United States

Remember that what you've just read is more than advice—it's a roadmap, a toolkit, and a companion for your journey in the United States nursing profession. Whether you are a foreign-trained nurse stepping onto American soil for the first time or a local nurse looking to elevate your career, the path ahead is filled with both challenges and incredible opportunities.

**Embrace the Learning Curve**

Entering or advancing in the nursing profession in the U.S. can feel overwhelming at times. From understanding licensing requirements and navigating cultural differences to adapting to new healthcare systems, the learning curve is steep—but entirely conquerable. Patience, persistence, and a willingness to learn will serve as your greatest allies. Celebrate small victories, and remember that every shift, every patient encounter, and every new skill you master is a step toward excellence.

**Build Your Network**

Your professional network will be one of your most valuable resources. Connect with fellow nurses, mentors, and professional organizations. Engage in local and national nursing associations, attend workshops, and participate in continuing education.

Networking is not just about finding opportunities—it's about creating a community of support, advice, and shared experiences that will carry you through the highs and lows of your career.

### Invest in Growth

Your education and professional development do not end once you receive your license. Pursue certifications in specialties that excite you, explore advanced degrees if your career goals require them, and remain curious about emerging technologies and innovations in healthcare. The more you invest in your knowledge, the more doors will open—both in terms of career advancement and personal fulfillment.

### Maintain Balance

Nursing is demanding, both physically and emotionally. Never underestimate the importance of self-care, mental wellness, and setting boundaries. A well-balanced nurse is not only more effective professionally but also happier personally. Remember, thriving in nursing is about sustainable excellence—not burnout.

### Embrace Your Unique Perspective

As a foreign-trained nurse or a nurse with diverse experiences, you bring a unique perspective to your practice. Your cultural insight, resilience, and adaptability are invaluable in today's diverse healthcare environment. Let these qualities guide your interactions with patients, colleagues, and communities—you have something no one else can offer.

**Look Ahead with Confidence**

The U.S. nursing profession is full of potential. Hospitals, clinics, research institutions, and educational programs are seeking passionate, skilled, and compassionate nurses. The roadmap you hold is not a set of limitations—it is a launching pad. Trust yourself, embrace challenges as opportunities, and know that each day you step into your role, you are making a meaningful difference in lives across the nation.

Your next chapter begins now. Step forward with courage. Lean on your knowledge, your network, and your passion. Let your journey be defined not by the obstacles you face but by the care you give, the lives you touch, and the legacy you create as a nurse in the United States. Because at the end of the day, nursing is not just a profession—it's a calling. And your calling is waiting.

# Chapter 24: A Letter to Your Future Self – Stepping Boldly into Nursing in the U.S.

**Dear Nurse,**

As you close this book, take a moment to acknowledge how far you've already come. The journey to becoming a nurse, especially in a new country, is not an easy one. It demands courage, resilience, and an unwavering commitment to care. And yet, here you are, ready to step forward into a profession that is as challenging as it is extraordinary.

The road ahead will not always be smooth. You will face long nights, tough decisions, moments of self-doubt, and times when the system feels overwhelming. But remember this: every challenge is also an opportunity. Every difficult shift, every complex patient, every new procedure mastered—these are your building blocks. They are shaping you into the nurse the world needs: skilled, compassionate, and unshakably human.

Believe in the power of your story. Your journey, your background, your training, your experiences gives you a unique lens through which to view care. No one else can offer what you can. Your voice, your perspective, and your empathy are gifts that will touch countless lives.

Seek growth relentlessly. Learn, ask questions, pursue certifications, and embrace opportunities that stretch your abilities. Let curiosity be your compass and ambition your engine. But also honor yourself along the way. Rest when you need it, care for your mind and body, and protect the balance that allows you to give your best to others.

Connect with those around you—mentors, peers, and communities. Your journey is not meant to be walked alone. Build bridges, share knowledge, and let the support of others lift you during the hardest moments.

Above all, step forward with courage. There will never be a "perfect" time to leap into your dreams—there will only be the moment you decide to trust yourself and take the next step. That moment is now. The world is ready for your compassion, your dedication, and your brilliance.

So go—enter your future with confidence. Own your space in the nursing profession. Touch lives, inspire others, and never forget that every patient, every colleague, and every challenge you meet is an opportunity to shine. Your calling is waiting, and the world needs the nurse only you can be.

With unwavering belief in you,

**Your Future Self**

# Chapter 25: Advice from Other Foreign-Educated Nurses Who Have Walk This Path Before

**Wanda Rose, BSN, RN (transitioned from Guyana to the USA)**

*"I highly recommend prospective international nurses to seek mentorship from colleagues who have successfully navigated the transition to nursing practice in the United States. Their firsthand experience can provide invaluable insights and practical guidance. Prior to leaving home, ensure that you designate a reliable and trustworthy individual to assist with critical administrative tasks, such as submitting payments to the necessary department personnel, in securing a smooth transition of your RN transcript to the US. Begin preparing for the NCLEX-RN exam well in advance of your arrival. Early study not only enhances your chances but also eases the adjustment process once in the US. And lastly, maintain an open and flexible mindset regarding a nursing specialty. Explore various fields, and identify one that aligns with your passion and strengths, and begin focusing your efforts in that direction. Clarifying your professional interest early will better equip you to adapt to the clinical and cultural environment of American healthcare."*

**Rhea Downer, MSN, RN, CMN (Nurse Tutor/ lecturer from Guyana) transitioned from Guyana to the USA**

*"Fulfilling the American dream requires adaptation, as it often involves navigating unfamiliar social and professional systems and embracing change in order to seize opportunities.*

*If I were to start over, I would begin the documentation process prior to migrating, as it would save time during the transition into specific roles.*

*Keep in mind that certificates obtained primarily in the United States are generally well-recognized and highly regarded.*

*When considering career advancement, focus on less popular programs that increase your marketability. Put God first while staying focused on long-term goals."*

**Jonna Alferez-Cordero, BSN, RN (transitioned from the Philippines to the USA)**

*"Do the required training, certifications and classes, have an open mind, seek every opportunity to learn and don't be afraid to ask questions and ask for help. Consider having experienced nurses as mentors to help navigate and better understand the dynamics of nursing and healthcare in the US."*

**Olivia Trotman Beharry, RN- best graduating Registered Nurse 2017 (Charles Rosa School of Nursing). transitioned from Guyana to the USA**

*"Financial Resources and faith and patience the size of a coconut and family support and this amazing book you will be the key to navigate the transition process smoothly.*

*1. Research and decide which U.S. state you want to live and work in. Visit the Board of Nursing (BON) website for that state to understand specific licensing requirements. Example: Florida BON, New York BON, Texas BON, etc. Each state may have slightly different requirements.*

*2. Since, you're coming from Guyana, CGFNS (Commission on Graduates of Foreign Nursing Schools) is the most recommended agency.*

***CGFNS evaluates:***

- *Education (transcripts, curriculum)*
- *License (status, history)"*
- *English proficiency (if applicable)*

*Below is a list of common costs associated with the transition process:*

- ***CGFNS Account Creation*** *→ Initial registration fee for evaluation service*

- ***Academic Report Processing Fee*** *→ Paid to your nursing school in Guyana for transcripts/documents*
- ***Guyana Nursing Council Fee*** *→ For license proof*
- ***CGFNS Reactivation Fees*** *→ If your license is inactive or outstanding balances are due*
- ***Document Shipping Fees*** *→ For CGFNS and State BON submissions*
- ***State Board of Nursing Application Fee*** *→ BON-specific licensing application charges*
- ***Required Courses (if needed)*** *→ e.g., CPR Certification, Infection Control*
- ***NCLEX Exam Fee*** *→ To sit for the NCLEX-RN*
- ***Other Hidden Costs*** *→ Background checks, fingerprinting, translations, etc.*

***Additional Steps You May Need***

- *English Language Proficiency Exam (not required for Guyana or English-speaking countries) – some states or CGFNS might require it.*
- *VisaScreen Certificate – required if you plan to immigrate to the U.S. to work as a nurse.*
- *NCLEX-RN Exam – Once your documents are approved, you'll need to pass this U.S. licensure exam.*

***Final Tip***

- *Keep multiple copies of all official documents.*

- *Start the process early – it can take several months, 6–12 months (mine took less than 6 months)*
- *Stay in touch with CGFNS (they reply fast and are always available on the phone to assist) and your chosen State BON for updates.*
- *Use a credit card or other trackable method for payments and keep receipts.*

*Hope these little tips help."*

**Maria, BSN RN from the Philippines**

*"Every challenge you face is a step toward becoming a stronger nurse. Don't rush—learn the system, ask questions, and trust your instincts."*

**Ahmed, RN from Egypt**

*"Coming to the U.S. as a foreign nurse can feel overwhelming, but patience and persistence pay off. Focus on one milestone at a time—NCLEX first, then experience, then growth."*

**Priya, RN CNM from India**

*"Your cultural background is your strength, not a weakness. Use your unique perspective to connect with patients and stand out as a compassionate caregiver."*

**Juan, RN from Mexico**

*"Networking is as important as studying. Talk to other nurses, join online forums, and don't hesitate to ask for guidance—it's how you learn the unwritten rules of nursing in the U.S."*

**Liana, RN from Russia**

*"Language and communication may feel like barriers at first, but clarity comes with practice. Don't be afraid to repeat, ask for clarification, or use your voice confidently."*

**Samuel, BSN RN from Ghana**

*"Every hospital, every unit is different. Be flexible, observe carefully, and adapt. Your willingness to learn will open doors faster than anything else."*

**Fatima, BSN RN from Pakistan**

*"Mistakes happen to everyone. What matters is how you respond. Own your learning, seek feedback, and use every experience as a stepping stone."*

**Thabo, RN from South Africa**

*"Never compare your journey to someone else's. Some paths are longer, some shorter, but every path leads to growth and opportunities in nursing."*

**Sofia, BSN RN from Brazil**

*"Invest in yourself—study, certifications, workshops. Knowledge builds confidence, and confidence builds respect in any workplace."*

**Hana, RN from Japan**

*"Remember why you became a nurse in the first place. Amid paperwork, long shifts, and challenges, your passion for helping people will guide you."*

# Chapter 26: Transition Checklist for Foreign-Educated Nurses in the USA

Here's a final reminder of the step-by-step transition checklist for foreign-educated nurses coming to the U.S. It's broken down into Before Arrival, Upon Arrival, First 6 Months, and First Year so it feels practical and easy to follow.

**Before Arrival**

**1. Licensure & Credentialing**

- Apply for credential evaluation (CGFNS, ERES, Josef Silny, or state-required body).
- Verify your nursing license with your home country board. Ensure your license is active (not expired) during the credential verification process.
- Register and prepare for the NCLEX-RN exam.
- Review state-specific requirements (each Board of Nursing has different rules).

**2. Immigration & Employment**

- If necessary, secure a work visa (commonly H-1B, TN, or EB-3) or green card sponsorship (not required for permanent residents or U.S. citizens).
- Research recruitment agencies or direct hospital employment.

- Collect and organize important documents (passport, transcripts, diplomas, immunization records).

**3. Preparation & Readiness**

- Improve English proficiency (especially medical terminology and communication skills).
- Familiarize yourself with U.S. healthcare practices (HIPAA, patient safety standards).
- Build a budget plan (moving expenses, initial housing, transportation).

**Upon Arrival**

**4. Practical Settling**

- Open a bank account.
- Apply for a Social Security Number (SSN).
- Get a U.S. phone number and internet service.
- Find housing (short-term or long-term).

**5. Employment Onboarding**

- Attend hospital orientation.
- Learn to use electronic health records (EHRs).
- Review facility protocols (medication administration, infection control).

**6. Healthcare & Insurance**

- Enroll in health insurance through your employer.

- Identify a primary care provider for yourself.

**First 6 Months**

**7. Workplace Adjustment**

- Build confidence in patient-centered communication.
- Understand nurse-patient ratios and workplace expectations.
- Learn about continuing education units (CEUs) and renewal deadlines.

**8. Professional Growth**

- Join nursing associations (ANA, state-level groups, minority nurse associations).
- Seek a mentor or preceptor for guidance.
- Consider specialty certifications if interested (BLS, ACLS, PALS, etc.).

**9. Cultural Adaptation**

- Learn U.S. workplace culture (teamwork, autonomy, direct communication).
- Be aware of possible microaggressions and learn how to self-advocate professionally.
- Connect with foreign nurse support groups for encouragement.

**First Year**

**10. Professional Development**

- Renew your nursing license if required.

- Take continuing education courses.
- Explore career advancement options (charge nurse, specialty training, advanced degrees).

**11. Financial Stability**

- Understand taxes, retirement plans (401k/403b), and credit scores.
- Create a savings plan for family, education, or future investments.

**12. Work-Life Balance**

- Adjust to 12-hour shifts and establish self-care routines.
- Build a healthy support system (friends, family, colleagues).
- Celebrate your milestones and achievements.

www.ingramcontent.com/pod-product-compliance
Lightning Source LLC
La Vergne TN
LVHW051045210926
848486LV00001B/25